Traditional Medicine in a Mediterranean Island Community

Charles Savona-Ventura

2021

Published by Lulu Press Inc., U.S.A.
ISBN: 978-1-68474-441-1

2

Contents

Introduction

Evidence-based medical practice is one of the buzzwords of modern medicine. Evidence-based medicine is defined as the reliance of available best evidence in making judicious and reasonable decisions relating to the care of individual patients. It does not allow for empirical observations but is very much dependent on systematic reviews and meta-analyses whereby physicians can identify the best studies related to a topic and critically analyse them to identify the best available mode of management.[1]

Traditional or Folk medicine refers to medical aspects of traditional knowledge related to heath care that developed over time within various communities before the era of modern medicine. It was more likely to be empirical and observational, often based on the passed down traditions of the senior members of the physician community. While the armamentarium of observational management options often had elements that afforded effective treatment; other treatments would in themselves be ineffective and potentially harmful. The World Health Organization (WHO) defines traditional medicine as 'the sum total of the knowledge, skills, and practices based on the theories, beliefs, and experiences indigenous to different cultures, whether explicable or not, used in the maintenance of health as well as in the prevention, diagnosis, improvement or treatment of physical and mental illness'.[2]

Traditional medical practices vary from one country to another, these being very often dependent on the cultural history of that country or region. The accumulation of the medical armamentarium of traditional medicine is strongly influenced by religious-superstitious and observational elements. This was eventually, mainly after the Classical Period, tempered by philosophical-rational concepts that opened the way

---

[1] I. Masic, M. Miokovic, B. Muhamedagic Evidence Based Medicine – New Approaches and Challenges. Acta Inform Med. 2008; 16(4):219–225

[2] WHO. The WHO Traditional Medicine Strategy 2014–2023. WHO, Geneva, 2014

to scientific-based medicine based on a deeper understanding of the pathophysiology of disease states.

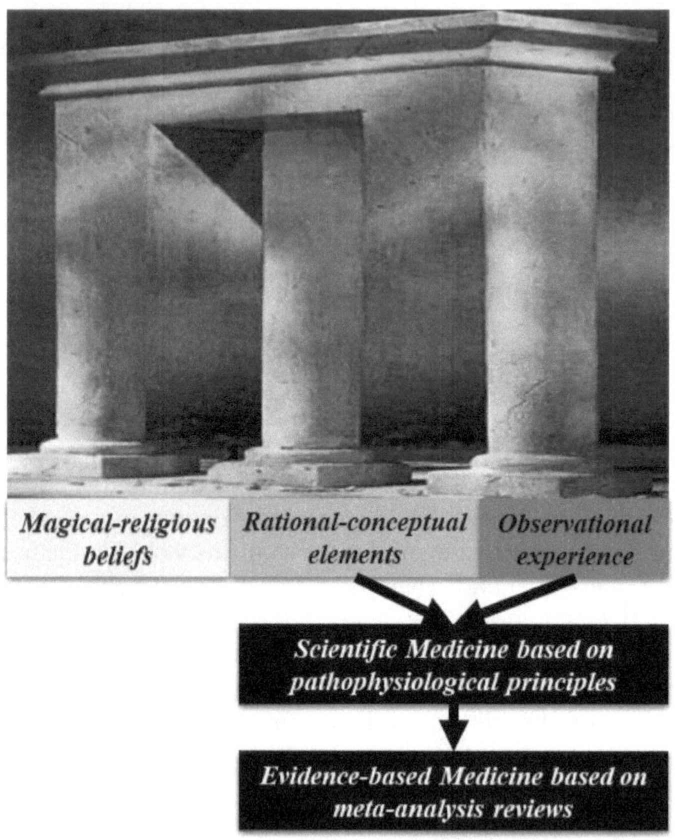

The development of traditional medical practices in any culture can be subdivided into three broad categories. These include practices that are primarily dependent on magic, superstition and religion grouped as magico-superstitious; practices based on observational study; and practices based on the rationalization of the aetiology of disease. The latter two practices can be said to have promoted the move towards the scientific understanding of disease processes and management to what can be considered modern evidence-based medicine. The actual practice of traditional medicine would therefore have both prophylactic and therapeutic elements involving lifestyle advice, physical interventions, and traditional medicinal products general herbal. The study of traditional medicine, in communities where this has fallen to the wayside, must be based on a study of folklore beliefs and popular proverbs, cognitive archaeology, and old texts.

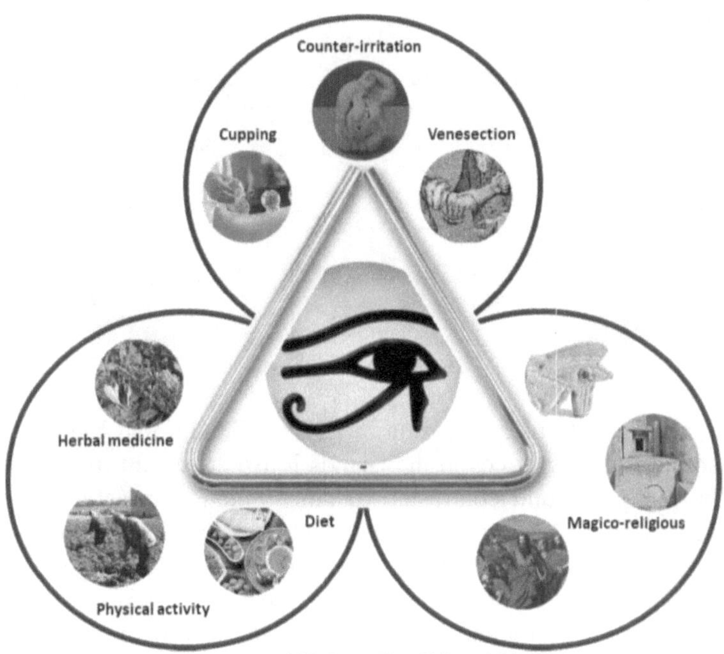

Components of Maltese Traditional Medicine

The Maltese Archipelago occupies a central position in the Mediterranean being hardly 93 kilometres away from Sicily and 290 km from Northern Africa. Gibraltar is 1836 km to the west and Alexandria is 1519 to the east. This central position within the Mediterranean Sea made the Islands an important meeting place for the various Mediterranean cultures throughout the ages merging and amalgamating European traditions with cultures derived from the Eastern Mediterranean lands and the Maghreb region of North Africa.

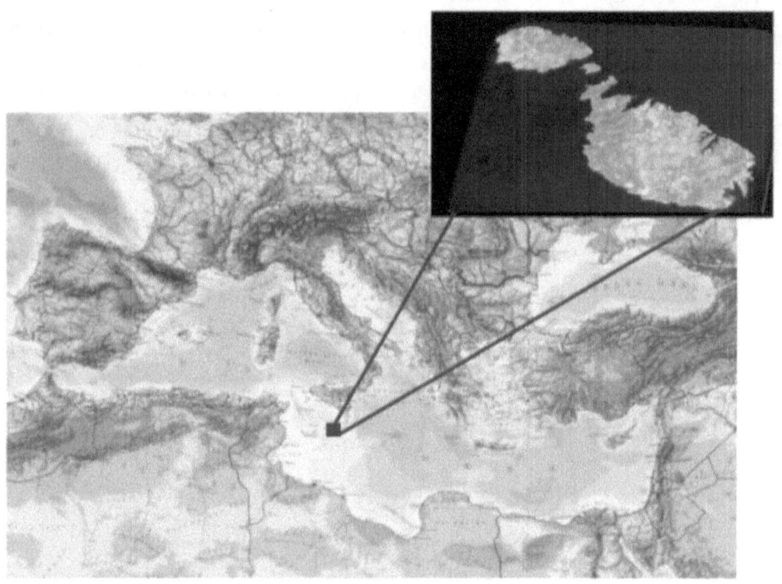

The Maltese Archipelago

For an adequate understanding of Maltese Traditional Medicine, one must not consider practices in the islands in isolation, but these practices must be compared and contrasted to other practices practiced in other countries in the Mediterranean basin. Maltese traditional medicine is based on a clash of cultures bringing together the different geographical regions [East-West-North-South], the European with African continents, and the Semitic to Islam and Christian cultures. An obvious mythological link promoting wellbeing from a North African culture can be seen in the decoration of the traditional Maltese fishing boats which often include the 'eye of Horus' placed there with the aim of protecting the fishermen working the boat.

Horus, son of Isis and Osiris, was the falcon-headed sky deity. The mythical story of his fight with Seth, established Horus as the deity of the sun and the deity of life and of all what was good. During his battle against Seth, Horus has his eye gouged out. This was later restored by the deity Thoth. The eye of Horus (the Ugiat) remained a magical talisman for health throughout Egyptian history. There have also been several

8

amulets depicting the Ugiat and of Horus excavated from various sites in Malta and Gozo.[3]

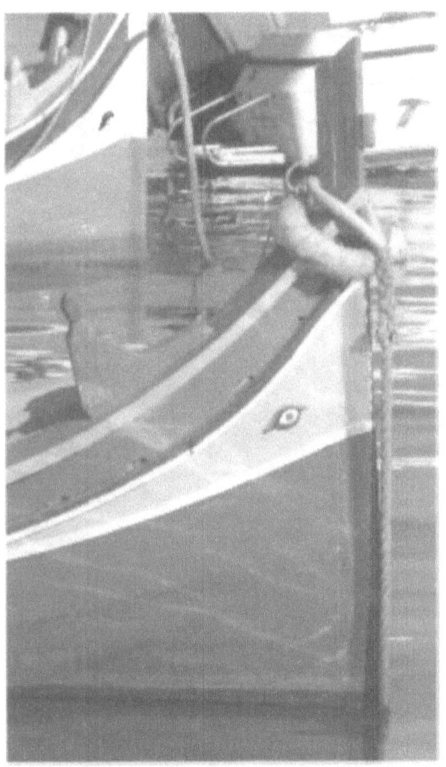

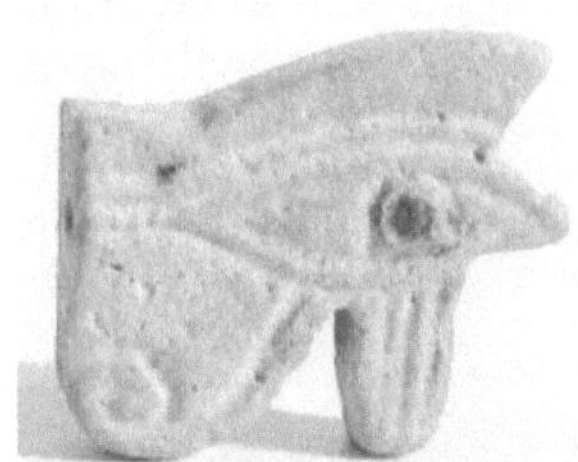

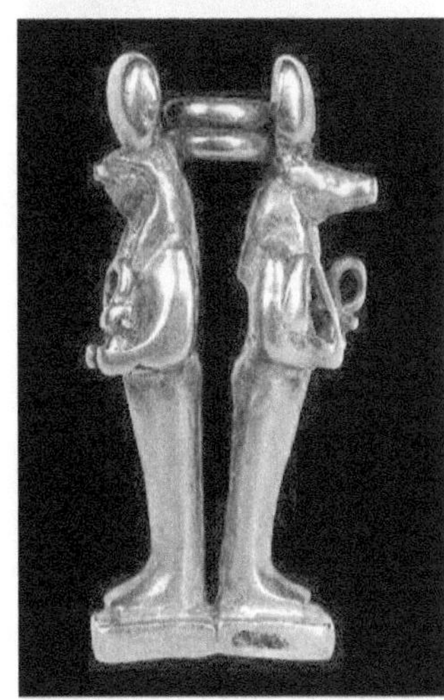

Maltese fishing boats with the Ugiat depicted at the bow	Archaeological artefacts depicting the Ugiat and Horus/Anubis

The medical historical heritage of the Maltese Islands can be traced back as far as man has been recorded to inhabit the Islands. Items related to what can be considered magico-religious medicine have been

---

[3] T. Gouder: Fuq xi Amuleti minn Malta Fenicjo-Punika. In: T. Cortis (ed.) Oqsma tal-Kultura Malitja. Kungress Nazzjonali 18-19 ta' April 1991. Malta: Ministry of Education, 1991, 67-82

excavated from several prehistoric sites in Malta and Gozo. Later period archaeological remains have also shown a continuing belief in the magico-religious, though with the emphasis being shifted to different deities. On another level, plant remedies have been resorted to since time immemorial with some of the early traditions persisting to date; while the corpus of traditional proverbs give remedies promoting a healthy wellbeing.

Magico-Religious Medicine

Introduction

Mythology or religious belief attempts to give an explanation of life-event uncertainties like failing crops, life, disease and death. These life-event problems are to the primitive non-scientific mind difficult to explain. Magico-religious or superstitious beliefs imply a belief in supernatural forces or beings who are both different and superior to living men in that they directly or indirectly exercise a benign or harmful influence. It is the function of ritual practices or ceremonies to encourage the former influence and prevent or neutralize the latter. Supernatural beings, the objects of these beliefs, can be divided into two categories. On the one hand there are the dead ancestors or manes who have been known to their contemporaries while alive; while on the other hand, there are the divinities who never existed as ordinary mortals.

The study of prehistoric mythology is frequently cited as a neglected, even dangerous area of archaeological study. Cognitive archaeology - the study of past ways of thought from material remains - is in many respects one of the newer branches of modern archaeology. The religions and myths of many prehistoric societies can only be gleaned through the interpretation of either physical traces of what appears to be vestiges of ritual practice or else pictorial representations of such practices from which can be inferred, with the aid of ethnological parallels, a belief in the existence of the supernatural beings to whom they were addressed. One cannot, therefore, insist too strongly on the hypothetical character of conclusions based on such material.[1]

Man is equipped with instincts that drive him to commit actions tending to preserve the individual, to propagate his kind, and to omit actions inimical to such a purpose. We may readily assume that man's

---

[1] C. Renfrew, P. Bahn. Archaeology. Theories, Methods and Practice. London: Thames and Hudson, 1994, 339-370

instincts were the purer the less developed his civilization was, i.e. the less his actions were the result of reflexes conditioned by a more complicated social environment. The main concern of prehistoric man and primitive human societies is that of survival and thus the procurement of an adequate daily diet. Major life events notably that of the delivery of a new-born in the community, the occurrence of disease, and the death of an individual were also important landmarks. It is not surprising that these four events - fertility, food procurement, illness, and death - were in many prehistoric and in primitive societies associated with magico-religious practices.

Medicine, magic and religion to primitive man were a set of practices intended to protect him against evil forces and spirits that inhabited his environment. The supernatural forces included the various deities and the ghosts of the dead which hovered over the village. In order to live safely, primitive man was required to be continuously on his guard to appease these supernatural forces. A serious illness was interpreted as being the result of an evil act performed either by a higher power, spirit, ghost or deity, in which case there was a religious explanation, or by a living person through sorcery, in which case there was a magical explanation. Sickness was induced either by the magical introduction of something foreign to the body (a "magic shot") or by the magical removal of a vital part or the soul. The magic shot generally explained acute painful illness that befalls the patient suddenly, while the loss of the soul or vital force was often held responsible for chronic disease where the patient slowly withered away.

The management of magico-religious disease states was based on efforts at prevention by undertaking continuing efforts at appeasing and warding off the deities, spirits, or ghosts of the dead; and in the presence of illness by the use of magical rites through the intervention of a medicine-man or shaman.[2]

---

[2] R. Porter. What is disease? In. R. Porter (ed.) The Cambridge Illustrated History of Medicine. Cambridge: University Press, 1996, 83-117

Appeasing the deities

Health and wellbeing are very much dependent on an adequate supply of food for the individual and the community. Linking the seasonal provision of food to the benevolence of a fertility deity, prehistoric man developed rites to appease the deity and earn its good will and providence. This magico-religious concept of a fertility deity in Europe became established during the Palaeolithic period. In the Maltese Islands, it became the central cult during the Neolithic period after the advent of farming and husbandry. Man the Farmer was very much concerned with survival and very conscious of the cyclical process of reproduction of his crops and stock, and of his own species. He believed that his survival depended on the fertility deity who regularly supplied him with his dietary requirements. This deity had to be regularly appeased to ensure its benevolence.[3]

The earliest accepted date for the presence of Neolithic Man in the Maltese Islands has been set by calibrated radiocarbon dating at circa 7,000 years ago which fits the time scale of the spread of early farming in Europe. Stone Age man in Malta thus appeared to have developed at circa 4400-4100 BCE (Before Common Era) a fertility cult in an effort to promote and encourage the reproductive cycle. What survives of this initial cult are the figurative representations around which these rites took place. These include the small fragmentary statuettes, which appear to emphasize the female sexual characteristics, and rubbed down animal bones which have been interpreted as phallic symbols.[4] By the fourth millennium BCE, the agricultural population was gradually set on a path of very independent cultural development - the Temple Period circa 4100-2500 BCE - which included active preventive efforts at appeasing the fertility deities represented principally by the megalithic temple structures and by the vestiges of items possibly used during the ritual practices.

---

[3] S. Stoddart, A. Bonanno, T. Gouder, C. Malone, D. Trump. Cult in an Island Society: Prehistoric Malta in the Tarxien Period. Cambridge Archaeological Journal, 1993, 3(1): 3-19; C. Renfrew. Before Civilization. The Radiocarbon revolution and prehistoric Europe. London: Penguin Books, 1973, 166-174

[4] D.H. Trump. Skorba. Excavations carried out on behalf of the National Museum of Malta 1961-1963. London: University Press, 1966, 33

The megalithic buildings of the Temple Period community in Malta have been associated with a progressive Fertility Cult on the basis of the clay statuettes and symbols associated with the fertility. Images of obese human deities said to represent the Mother Earth deity, similar to those excavated from Malta, have been described from the Upper Palaeolithic era (about 25000 years ago) to the dawn of metal-using European societies in the Neolithic era. A few have been found in Western Europe, but the yields have been much richer at sites in Egypt, the Levant, Turkey, Greece, Cyprus and the Balkans.[5] Animal bas reliefs in the various temples, particularly the bull associated with the cow and her thirteen young sucklings at Tarxien Temples, are further strongly suggestive of fertility magic. The Tarxien Temple bas relief bovid couple are similar in style to Palaeolithic ones described from Le Fourneau du Diable and Levanzo.[6] In the Maltese context, the Fertility deity may have not been restricted to one deity but rather a trinity of deities explaining the discovery of statuettes showing three figures from Xghara Circle and Hagar Qim, and possibly the three temple groups at Mnaidra and Hagar Qim.

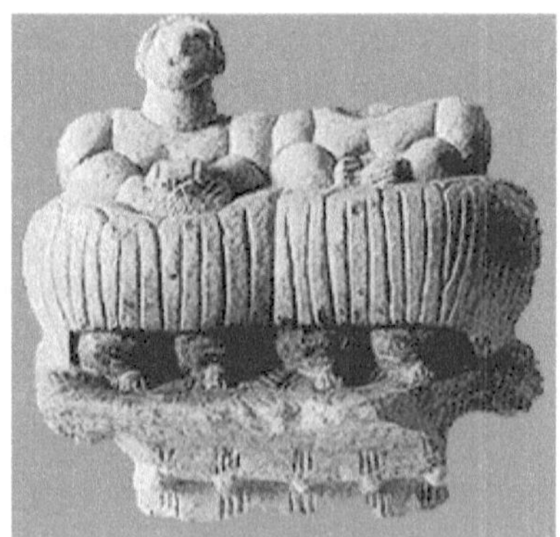

Fertility trinity
Xghara Circle

---

[5] V. Veen. The goddess of Malta. The lady of the Waters and the earth. Holland: Inanna-Fia Publ, 1992

[6] A, Mifsud, S. Mifsud. Dossier Malta: Evidence for the Magdalenian. Malta: Proprint, 1997, 144-145

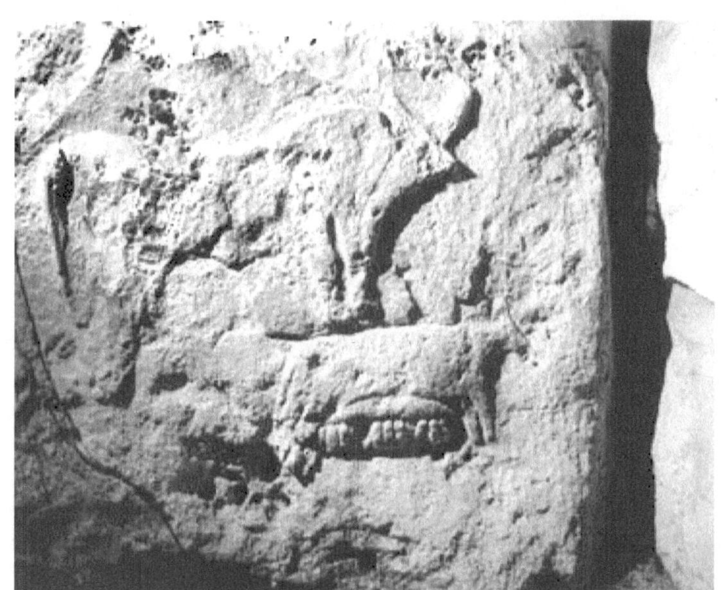

**Coupling bull and cow with young
Tarxien Temples**

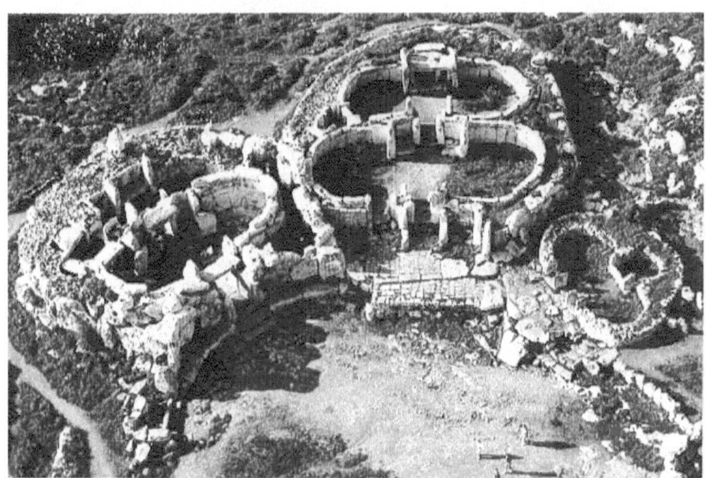

**Ggantija group of three temples complex with a human form
suggesting a belief of entering back into Mother Earth for protection**

In a society in which the family had to be supported by the labour and produce of its members, the birth of a child must have been an important and special event in the lives of the family group and the community, a special gift to the community from the Mother earth deity. Three small clay statuettes, from Mnaidra Temple, Tarxien Temple and the Hal Saflieni Hypogeum, represent a female body with a great projecting abdomen, large breasts and very detailed representation of the vertebrae and ribs. In the specimens from Mnaidra and Tarxien the genitalia are well illustrated. Posteriorly the figures are represented as wasted, and the iliac regions represented as hollow. The back in the Tarxien specimen has a kyphotic curve. The latter also has a number of fragments of shell stuck symmetrically into different parts. It has been suggested that these two specimens may represent an abdominal tumour, ascites or filariasis, while the shell fragments may reflect the use of witchcraft or counter-irritation.[7] In the presence of a fertility cult, the grossly enlarged abdomen, the pendulous breasts and the emphasized genital features of these figurines most likely depict a pregnancy state and may be examples of sympathetic magic related to fertility. The incisional marks on the back on two of these statuettes can be interpreted as depicting the lunar months of pregnancy.

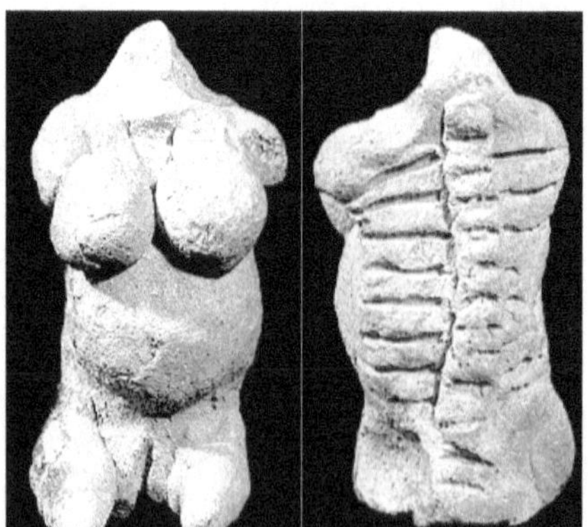

Pregnant woman - Mnaidra temple

---

[7] T. Ashby. Supplementary excavations at Hagar Kim and Mnaidra in June 1910. Archivum Melitense 1910, 1(2/3/4):59; T. Zammit, C. Singer. Neolithic representations of the human form from the Islands of Malta and Gozo. J Roy Anthrop Instit, 1924, 54:92,96

The ritual practices in these "temples" apparently included the ritual sacrifice of domesticated animals and collected foodstuff such as fish and seashells. This is evidenced by the finds at the Tarxien Temples wherein a sacrificial altar with a curved flint knife in its interior was described. At the same temple complex several animal depictions showing the ibex, mouflon, pig, bull and cow were described, while several seashells were also found. Fish depictions were recorded from the Bugibba Temple.[8] Presumably the ritual sacrifice would also have included agricultural products, thus encompassing all the "gifts" of the Mother Earth deity. There is no archaeological evidence that human sacrifice was practiced during this phase of Maltese prehistory.

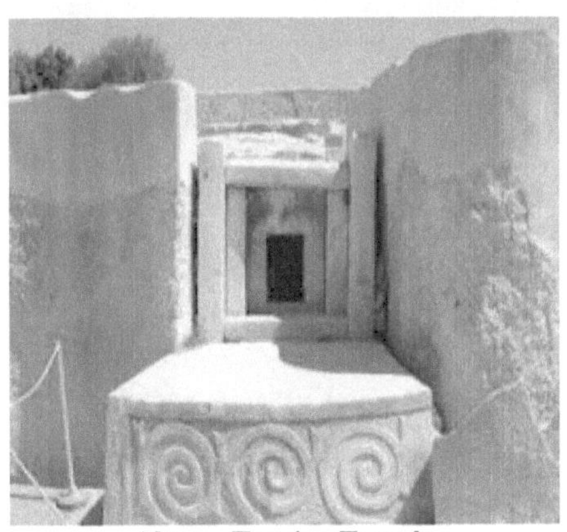

Altar – Tarxien Temple

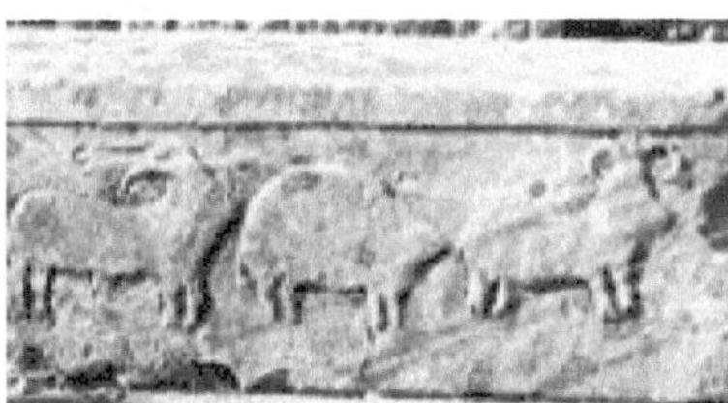

Ibis – Pig – Mouflon
Tarxien Temples

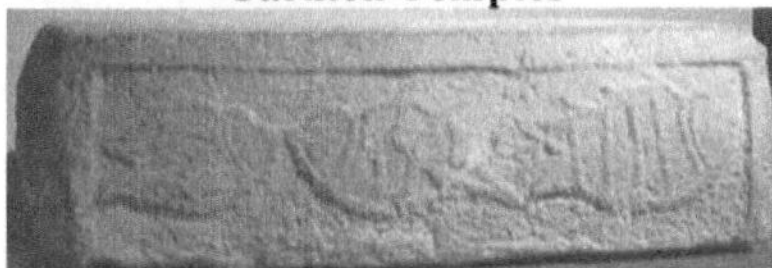

Fish
Bugibba Temple

The Temple Period society appears to have suddenly disappeared from the Islands at about 2100 BCE, to be eventually replaced by communities from the Aegean and the Eastern Mediterranean. In the first millennium BCE, the Maltese inhabitants established trade and cultural links with the Phoenicians who originally inhabited the eastern shores of the Mediterranean to the north of Mount Carmel, between Palestine and Syria. These were seafarers who plied their trade throughout the

---

[8] J.D. Evans. The Prehistoric Antiquities of the Maltese Islands: A Survey. London: Athlone Press, 1971, 116-149, 109-112

Mediterranean establishing a western colony of Carthage in North Africa. Carthage dominated the western Mediterranean until the city was finally destroyed by the Romans in 146 BCE.[9] The Semitic Period of Maltese history [700-218 BCE] saw the assimilation of the pantheon of Semitic deities by the Maltese inhabitants, including the deity responsible for fertility and providence of food.

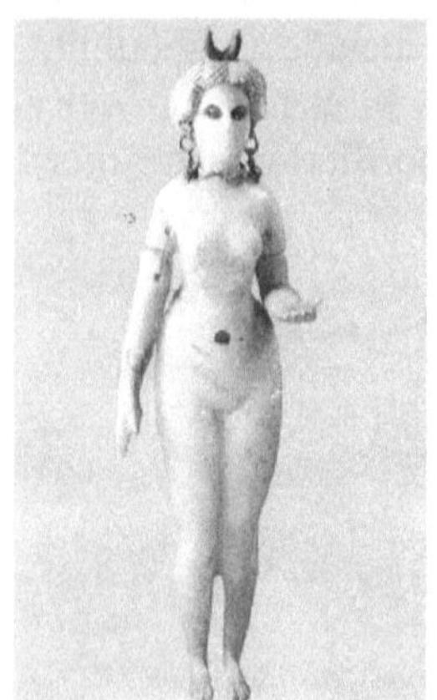
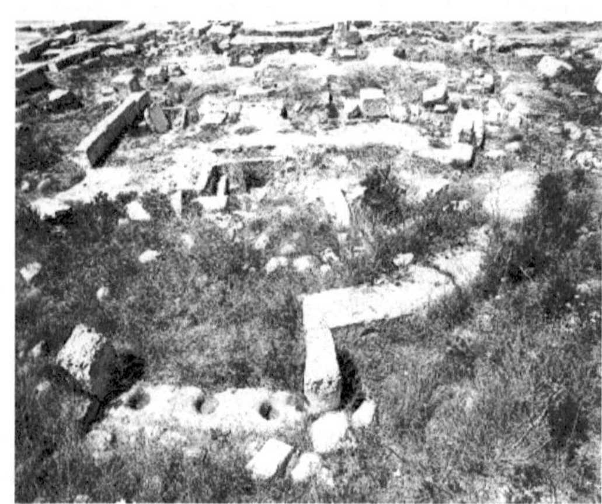

Astrate – Tas-Silg Temple remains

Ptolemy described a sanctuary dedicated to the female divinity Astarte, known also as Ashtar, Ishtar (to the Babylonians), Ashtoreth (to the Hebrews), Tanit (to the Carthaginians) and Juno (to the Romans). This sanctuary was also mentioned by Cicero. The locality of this sanctuary has now been established at Tas-Silg at Marsaxlokk, Malta where excavations carried out by the Italian Archaeological Mission from the University of Rome in the 1960's revealed several scores of inscriptions invoking the goddess. Astarte was the goddess of fertility of the Semitic races. Her domain embraced all nature, vegetable and animal

---

[9] H. Bondi, A. Bullock, W. Gordon, D. Piper, B. Williams (eds): The Mind Alive Encyclopedia. Early Civilization. London: Marshall Cavendish Books Ltd., 1977, 33-36

as well as human. Afterwards she became the goddess of love in its noblest aspect as well as in its most degraded.[10]

The Islands remained under Carthaginian rule until they were included under Roman dominion in 218 BCE, though, in line with the generally tolerant policy towards the cultures of the subjected states, no pressure was made by the new rulers to undermine the Punic culture of the Maltese inhabitants and for a couple of centuries the Punic substratum can be detected in the archaeological record.[11] The Maltese community was introduced with Christianity in 60 ACE (After Common Era) with the arrival of the apostle Saul/Paul on the islands. This religion took a definite hold in the community after the fourth century ACE. The new deity was thus attributed with overreaching powers of reward and punishment of the individual and the community. He was the provider of all that was essential for man's survival.

The concept of appeasing and asking for God's provision of nutritional resources and hence ensure the fertility of the land is addressed within the Christian Calendar of events. Rogation Sunday falling on the first Sunday of May traditionally provides for a procession round the parish and the blessing of the crops and animals of the community. Rogation, meaning 'to ask', refers to the liturgical reading of the day which includes the words 'whatever you ask the Father in my name, he will give you'.[12] Another similar traditional feast practiced in Malta is the feast of *Imnaria* commemorating the Feast of the two

---

[10] T.C. Gouder, 1978: op. cit.; A. Bonanno, 1982: op. cit.; J. Quintin d'Autun: Insulae Melitae Descriptio, Lyons, 1536 (facsimile ed. Malta: Bibliotheca), 3-4; H.C.R. Vella: The earliest description of Malta (Lyons 1536). Translation and Notes. Malta: DeBono Enterprises, 1980, 20-23; G.F. Abela: Della descrittione di Malta isola nel Mare Siciliano con le sue antichita'. Malta; Paolo Bonacota, 1647 (facsimile ed. Malta: Midsea Books, 1984), 154-157; O. Bres: Malta Antica Illustrata co' Monumenti e coll'Istoria. Rome: Stamperia De Romanis, 1816 (facsimile ed. Malta: Midsea Books, 1986), 70-147

[11] T.C. Gouder: Phoenician Malta. Heritage. An Encyclopædia of Maltese Culture and Civilization, 1978, 1:173-186; T.C. Gouder: Some amulets from Phoenician Malta. Heritage. An Encyclopædia of Maltese Culture and Civilization, 1978a, 1:311-315

[12] The New Testament - English Standard Version. John, Chap 16, verse 23

apostles St. Peter and St. Paul held on the 29th of June. This event is a typical Maltese folklore harvest festival with plenty of music, folk dancing, feasting and colourful horses and donkey races at Buskett Gardens at Rabat in Malta.

These beliefs are strongly in grained as evidenced by the wide corpus of Maltese proverbs dealing with providence.[13]

Alla jsebbaħ; Alla jibgħat	God bring the dawn; God provides
Afda f'Alla u tħabbilx rasek	Trust in God and do not worry
Alla jagħlaq bieb u jiftaħ mija (ieħor)	God shuts one door and opens a hundred (other)
Alla fettieħi u Alla ħanin (għajur)	God is bountiful and God is merciful (jealous)
Alla jaħseb	God provides
Alla hu fuq kollox u kulħadd; xemx u xita jibgħat lil kulħadd	God is above everything and above all; sun and rain He sends for all.
Alla jara (jista') kollox	God sees (can do) everything

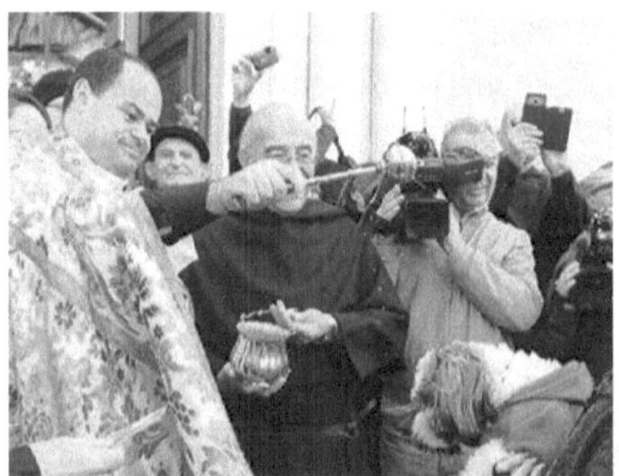

Rogation Sunday: Blessing of animals

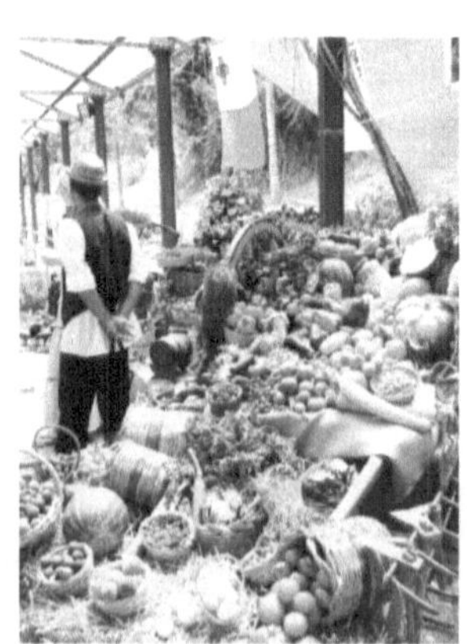

29th June: Imnarja

---

[13] J. Aquilina. A comparative dictionary of Maltese Proverbs. Malta: University Press, 1986.

Appeasing spirits of the dead

Other spirits considered to have supernatural powers needing appeasement are the spirits of the immediate dead who are believed to have the power to invade the living to perpetuate their existence. This fear was managed by the development of death cult rituals aimed at appeasing the dead ancestors and prevent their ghosts from causing harm to the community, particularly until the soul transgressed to the afterlife – in effect laying the dead spirit to rest. These death cult rituals date back to prehistory and up to present time. Palaeolithic man in Europe also took special concern with the burial of his dead, these being buried in the sleeping position, painted with red ochre to give the corpse a live appearance and decorated with necklaces or crowns of shells, with various implements placed beside them.[14] These Old Stone Age practices exemplify man's earliest preoccupation with the supernatural in his struggle for survival by ensuring appeasement of the dead ancestors. These death cult rituals are also evident throughout Maltese history.

Neolithic Man in Malta also took extreme efforts to appease the ghosts of the dead ancestors. It has been suggested that the development of the death cult in the Temple Period was related to the fertility cult and that the fertility deity had an interest in death as well as fertility, death being looked upon as a prelude to rebirth. The inclusion of grave good during burial is sometimes assumed to indicate a belief in an afterlife, but this need not necessarily follow. In some societies, the deceased's treasured possessions are so firmly associated with him or her that for another to own them would bring ill luck, and there is therefore a need to dispose of them with the dead, rather than for the future use of the dead. Because of the adopted custom of reburial of skeletal remains (*scarnitura*), it is to be expected that prehistoric man during the Temple Period in Malta was well aware of the destructibility of the human form.[15] The ritual attention,

---

[14] G.H. Luquet. Prehistoric Mythology. In. R. Graves (ed.) New Larousse Encyclopedia of Mythology. London: Hamlyn, 1981, 1-8; P. Phillips. The Prehistory of Europe. London: Penguin Books, 1980, 141-146

[15] C. Malone, A. Bonanno, T. Gouder, S. Stoddart, D. Trump. The Death Cults of Prehistoric Malta. Scientific American. December 1995:76-83; C. Renfrew, P. Bahn, Archaeology. Theories, Methods and Practice. London: Thames and Hudson, 1994, 363

including the positioning in the foetal sleeping position and the red ochre wash, given to the dead at the primary burial probably served a different purpose than simply a belief in a physical rebirth. Rebirth was thus more probably looked upon as the birth of the spirit or soul in the afterlife. The aim of the death cult ritual was more probably to help lay the dead to rest and provide them with a life-like sleeping form for the spirit to inhabit.

The burial customs of the Early Neolithic farmers in Malta are still not established, though skeletal material possibly belonging to Early Neolithic man has been excavated from various sites in Malta and Gozo. This material however was frequently fragmented and afforded little information. Excavations in 1911 at Santa Verna in Gozo dated by pottery associations to circa 5000-4500 BCE, revealed two whole skeletons interred with a heap of human bones; these belonged to at least three persons buried in earth stained with red ochre. The adult skeleton was buried straight on the back with folded arms. It has therefore been suggested that these burials were from a later period than indicated by the shards since all previously discovered Neolithic burials were found in the flexed position.[16]

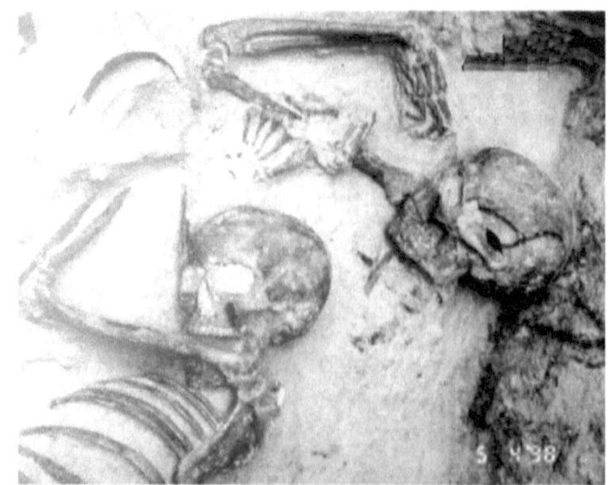

Temple Period articulated skeletons – Xghara Circle

---

[16] T. Zammit. The "Santa Verna" Neolithic Station. Reports on the Working of Government Departments during the financial year 1911-12. Malta: Government Printing Office, 1912, E1-E2; J.D. Evans. The Prehistoric Antiquities of the Maltese Islands: A Survey. London: Athlone Press, 1971, 188

The burial customs of Late Neolithic man of the Temple Period apparently progressed in line with the development of the above ground megalithic structures. The three-stage development first saw the introduction of the earliest rock-cut chamber tombs during the Zebbug Phase (circa 4100-3800 BCE). Recorded evidence shows that these monuments consisted of simple chambers that were accessed through a shaft. The second stage occurred during the Ggantija Phase, circa 3600-3000 BCE. This was characterized by a preference for larger facilities giving rise to collective burials, in contrast to the preceding simple rock-cut chamber tombs. This collective burial process gave rise to the third and final stage in the development of burial site typology which occurred during the Tarxien Phase, circa 3300-2500 BCE, at a time when the communal hypogea were embellished with rock carvings and ochre paintings. The three-stage development in burial facilities was a gradual one and often overlapped into different cultural pottery phases.[17] Hypogea are represented by Hal Saflieni Hypogeum, attributed to circa 3300-3000 BCE in Malta; and by the Xghara (also known as Brochtorff) Circle in Gozo, circa 4100-2500 BCE. Important cave-tombs in Malta include Gzibbu Tombs at Zebbug circa 4100-3800 BCE; Xemxija Tombs at St. Paul's Bay circa 3800-3600 BCE; and BurMghez Tombs at Mqabba circa 3600-3300/3000 BCE. Apart from the Xghara Circle, the dating of these burial sites has been based mainly on the associated pottery.

Man during the Temple Period in Malta buried his dead in the foetal or sleeping posture, interpreted as the desire to give the diseased an ideal resting position or as a preparation for a rebirth. The death bed was often covered with ochre, probably regarded as a replacement of blood for life hereafter. Red Ochre staining was noted at various Temple Period burial sites including the Buqana Rock Tomb, Hal Saflieni Hypogeum, Xaghra, Xghara Circle, and other sites. The primary burial rites evidently included the internment of gifts with the dead. These grave goods included pottery, stone axes, and shell, bone or stone bead pendants and necklaces. Sea-shells, such as those found at Zebbug, Xemxija and Pergla Tombs, have also been associated with life after death being symbolic of the vulva

---

[17] A. Pace. The Archaeology of collectivity. Cognitive Design Process: the case of Maltese prehistoric funerary sites (4000-2500 BC). Malta Archaeological Review 1997, 2:14-19

through which life was born. The burial sites were regularly visited and bones from earlier burials were progressively removed and stacked to allow space for later burials.[18]

The burial customs of Maltese Late Neolithic man were similar to those described elsewhere in Europe in inhumations dating as far back as the Palaeolithic period, with the placing of the dead in the foetal or sleeping position with the inclusion of grave goods, and the liberal covering of the dead with red ochre. The burial ritual may thus have served to mimic a comfortable rest. To most primitive people, the world of the dead is a very real one. The spirits of the ancestors are never far away and take an active part in life, bringing good and bad luck. At the point of death, when the soul leaves the body, the soul is not yet reconciled to its fate and may wish to come back to life by entering some other body thus causing illness. Particularly feared were the ghosts of people who died without having fulfilled their mission on earth - young children, brides, women in childbirth, etc. These more than any other dead would be eager to return to life or, feeling lonely, they may kill a close relative for company in the world of spirits.

Corpses were the object of practices which give evidence of deference and were buried with funerary intention. In many cases objects were placed with the bodies constituting funerary furnishings, while red ochre was sprinkled over the corpse in an attempt to strengthen and help the dead during the journey into the after-world.[19]

This concern with the disposal of the dead was carried through to the centuries. The Bronze Age Period was generally characterised by cremation practices whereby the dead body was burnt to ashes. This is clearly evident through the excavations carried out at the Tarxien Cemetery Phase. The source country of cremation development for the Bronze Age Mediterranean was most probably Anatolia. Cremation became the dominating burial custom near the end of the Late Bronze

---

[18] H.E. Sigerist. A History of Medicine. 1: Primitive and Archaic Medicine. New York: Oxford University Press, 1967, 106; Evans, 1971, 115, 167,186; Malone et al, 1993, 76-83
[19] Sigerist, 1967, 136-137

24

Age in Central Europe and Italy, and it also gained popularity in SyroPalestine. The practice was very well known there, especially in Central Europe, in the 3rd and 2nd millennia BCE. It arrived at Malta in the middle of the 2nd millennium, and in Magna Grecia it was sporadically practiced from the 15th century.[20]

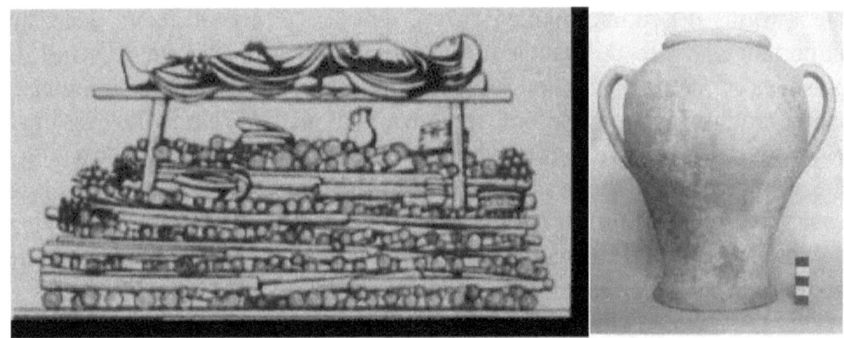

Cremation & Cinerary Urn, St Agatha Catacombs, Malta

The trade exposure to the Eastern Mediterranean introduced the Maltese inhabitants to the Semitic Phoenician culture. In Punic mythology, death was conceived as a supernatural power called Muth, but this deity was not worshipped and played no part in any Phoenician religious cult. The Phoenicians did however believe in an afterlife and in the long sea-voyage that led the deceased to the world of the dead. These beliefs are evidenced by the care given to their tombs containing grave-goods and the Egyptian-style talismans associated with death. A sixth century BC bronze amulet sheath containing a small rolled-up piece of papyrus bearing a Phoenician inscription with a representation to Isis was found in a tomb at Tal-Virtu, limits of Rabat, Malta. The sheath with a cover in the form of a falcon's head representing Horus - the Egyptian solar divinity - belongs to a distinct class manufactured in rigid imitation of Egyptian prototypes and widely diffused in Phoenicia and its colonies. The inscription has been translated to read *"laugh at your enemy O*

---

[20] K. Lewartowski. Cremation and the end of Mycenaean culture. Swiatowit, 1998, 41/Fac.A:136-145

valiant ones, scorn, assail and crush your adversary ......disdain (him), trample (him) on the waters; .....moreover prostate (him) .....on the sea, bind (him), hang (him)". These are the words of Isis - the sorrowing wife and eternal mother, protectress of the dead - addressed to the deceased and which ensured her assistance for an unfailing victory over a mythical adversary barring the way to the afterlife. Isis is in the papyrus represented bearing a throne upon her head, the ideogram of her name. In the various Egyptian medical texts, Isis is shown to have held an important place in the pantheon of healing deities. Her legend is full of episodes of magic cures, and repeatedly she appears as the great magician whose counsel is the breath of life, whose sayings drive out sickness, and whose word gives life to him whose breath is failing. Isis was adopted by the Romans when she was considered a healing goddess, discoverer of drugs, versed in the art of curing people who flocked to her temples, lying down in the halls, expecting to be delivered of their ailments by the goddess in their sleep.[21]

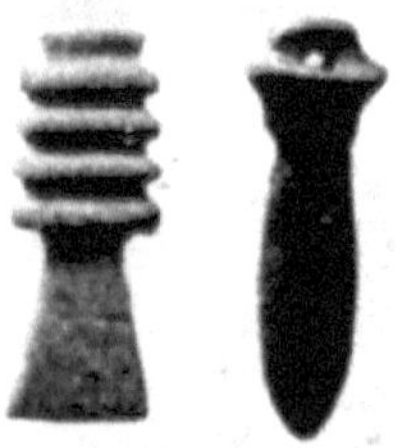

Dejd and Ouaz pillars – Malta

Related to the cult of the afterlife were faience amulets depicting the Djed and Ouaz pillars dated to the 7th-6th century BCE excavated from Bingemma near Rabat, Malta. The Djed pillar, symbol of stability, seemingly originated from the form of a column of bound papyrus was a simple fetish representing Osiris - god of the dead. Osiris gave his devotees the hope of an eternally happy life in another world ruled over

---

[21] T.C. Gouder, B. Rocco: Un talismano bronzeo da Malta contenente un nastro di papiro con iscrizione fenicia. Studi Magrebini, VII Napoli, 1975, 1-18; T.C. Gouder, 1978a: op. cit.; J. Viaud, 1981: op. cit.; E. Sykes, 1993: op. cit., 97-98; H.E. Sigerist, 1951: op. cit., 288

26

by a just and good king. The Ouaz pillar derived from the form of the lotus flower was the symbol of rebirth.[22]

Burial practices on the Maltese Islands developed in line with the prevalent religious beliefs throughout the centuries. The Punic tradition was maintained even during a large part of the Roman Empire dominion; however, the practice of cremation was subsequently re-introduced on the Islands during then later Roman Period Phase being practiced contemporaneously with inhumation practices. These tomb burials developed from isolated dug-out structures, to communal tombs and subsequently into large hypogea sited outside the walls of the cities or at a distance from the community. The burial of a loved one was a complex affair associated with a defined ritual at the time of death and a commemorative one in subsequent years. This ritual, aimed primarily at laying the dead the person to rest, was modified with the advent of Christianity and tied with the concept of resurrection even in the knowledge of the destructibility of the human form.

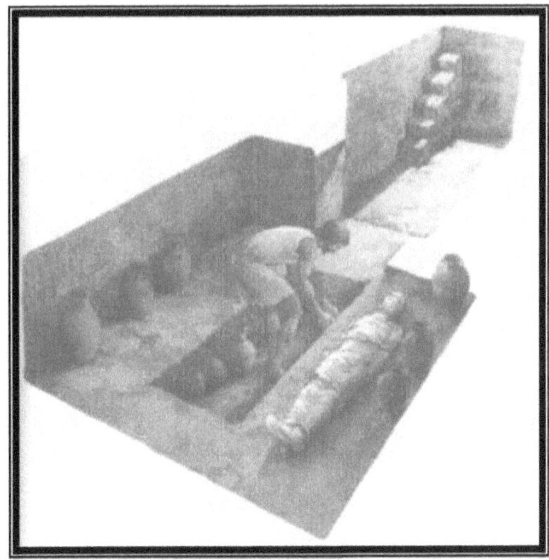

Punic burial

---

[22] T.C. Gouder, 1978a: op. cit.; J. Viaud, 1981: op. cit.

The advent of Christianity to the Islands, probably in the fourth century ACE, re-established the Semitic preference for inhumation with a complex dedicated ritual serving to put the dead to rest and helping the spirit soul of the dead to go to eternal life awaiting the eventual future resurrection of the physical body at the end of time. During the Medieval Period, preference was given to church burials thus placing the individual in a sanctified site. Concerns for hygiene in the nineteenth century led to the establishment of dedicated extensions of the formal religious establishments in the form of cemeteries. In modern times, the burial ritual remains a complex one intimately tied to the belief in an afterlife and a resurrection at the end of time. The ritual involves a dedicated religious ceremony with the presence of the deceased in his/her coffin. The ritual continues with the accompaniment of the deceased by the family members and friends to the gravesite where he/she is eventually buried. After the burial, the family members often congregate together in a home to reminisce about the decease and provide support to each other.

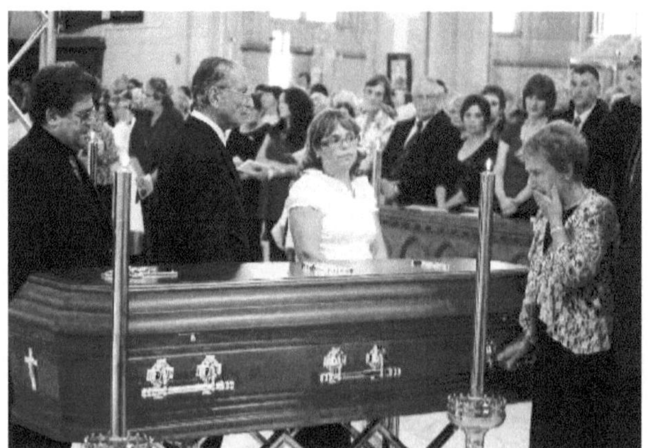

Burial ritual - Malta

28

Protection from Malevolent Spirits

Prehistoric man, like primitive man, believed that internal disease and death were brought on by malevolent spirits or enemy. He thus took precautions to ward off disease and evil spirits through the use of amulets. Amulets are objects that possess magical properties, and whose action is directed towards warding off evil or catching and neutralizing evil magic. There is an infinite variety of amulets, some of which can be distinguished into various groups. One group consists of objects having the faculty of inflicting wounds such as sharp and cutting objects, animal teeth and claws. A second group of amulets is represented by reproductions of the male and female genital organs and seashells whose life-bearing properties give protection. Other objects used as amulets include reproductions of the hand, foot, leg, heart, animals' eyes, and snake. Precious stones are also considered powerful amulets, their glittering attracting the evil eye, holding it and neutralizing it.[23]

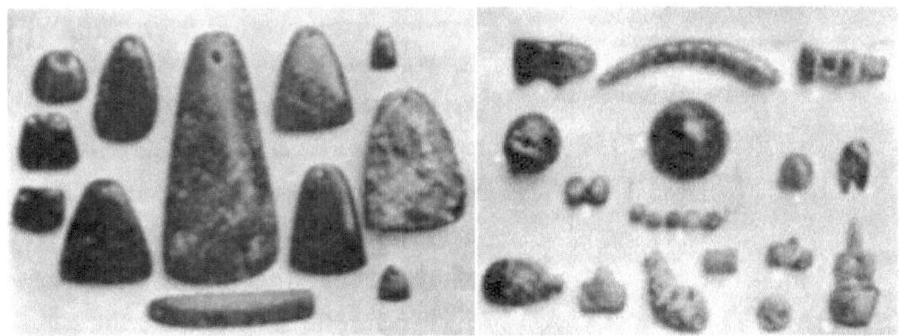

Neolithic amulets; Ghar Dalam, Malta

The use of amulets in Malta has apparently been in vogue since prehistoric times. A number of carved objects and statuettes excavated from Neolithic sites can be interpreted as having a protective function from evil magic. These included a number of personal ornaments incorporating seashells and fossilized shells, axe and tooth amulets, phallic symbols, and "Venus" figurines. The use of amulets to ward off

---

[23] C. Read. Man and his superstitions. London: Senate Books, 1995, 256-274; Sigerist, 1967, 144-146

evil continued to be used in later times with the advent of the Punic Semitic culture and persisted to until relatively recent times.[24]

Horus, son of Isis and Osiris, was the falcon-headed sky deity. The mythical story of his fight with Seth, established Horus as the deity of the sun and the deity of life and of all what was good. During his battle against Seth, Horus has his eye gouged out. This was later restored by the deity Thoth. The eye of Horus (the Ugiat) remained a magical talisman for health throughout Egyptian history. The British Museum Medical Papyrus written at the end of the XVIIIth Dynasty (circa 14th century BCE) records how the Ugiat was invoked while applying a remedy to diseased eyes with the following charm recited four times. *"This Eye of Horus created by the spirits of Heliopolis, which Thoth has brought from Hermopolis – from the great hall in Heliopolis, - in Pe,- in Dep, sayest thou to it: 'Welcome, thou splendid Eye of Horus, - thou content of the Eye of Horus – brought to drive out evil of the god, the evil of goddess, the demon, male and female, the dead, male and female, the enemy, male and female, who have insinuated themselves into the eyes of the sick under my fingers. – Protection, behind me protection, come protection!"* Horus had also been stung by a deadly scorpion and was saved by the powerful spells of the gods. He thus was considered to have himself acquired special facilities to cure people bitten by venomous animals. There have also been several amulets depicting the Ugiat excavated from various sites in Malta and Gozo (e.g. the faience amulets excavated from Tal-Horob, Xewkija, Gozo in 1951 dated c.5th-4th century BCE).

A gold amulet excavated from Ghajn Klieb, west of Rabat, Malta depicts the figure of falcon-headed Horus and jackal-headed Anubis. The two figures were in antiquity soldered together at the base and the top. In spite of their strikingly Egyptian appearance, the figures are considered to be very probably of eastern Phoenician manufacture. Anubis was the Egyptian deity who presided over the embalming of the dead. The name signifies watcher and guardian of the dogs. He presided over the abode of the dead, led the deceased to the judgement hall and supervised the weighing of the heart. Amulets depicting ibis-headed or dog-headed ape

---

[24] P. Cassar. The Medical History of Malta, London: Wellcome Historical Library, 1964, 421-436

30

Thoth have also been found in Maltese tombs. In the introduction to the Ebbers Papyrus, it is stated that "*I* (Re, the sun god) *will save him from his enemies, and Thoth shall be his guide, he who lets writing speak and has composed books; he gives to the skilful, to the physicians who accompany him, skill to cure.*" Thoth was considered a great physician and magician acting as physician to the god Horus. He was regarded as the god of magic and was the arbiter between the gods and had the knowledge needed by the dead to pass safely through the underworld.[25] In this pantheon of Egyptian deities, another respected deity was Isis, mother of Horus.

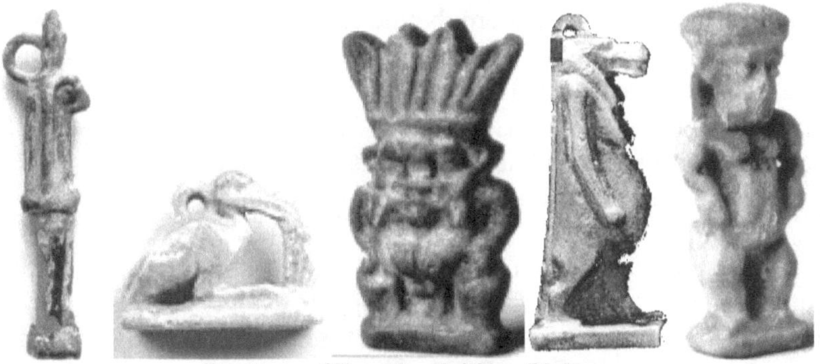

Pantheon of Egyptian deities – Malta
Horus, Thoth, Bes, Toueris, Ptah-Patecus

Further talisman in the form of faience amulet figurines representing Bes and Toueris have also been excavated from the Punic Period tombs. Bes, an African deity by origin, was a popular god known also in Egypt and western Asia. He was a frightening dwarf with bowlegs, a prominent belly, and an animal-like face with bulging eyes. He was frequently clothed with a panther skin with claws, sported a distinctive headdress, and wore a metal disc around his neck. This made him a veritable

---

[25] T.C. Gouder, 1978a: op. cit.; T. Gouder: Fuq xi Amuleti minn Malta Fenicjo-Punika. In: T. Cortis (ed.) Oqsma tal-Kultura Malitja. Kungress Nazzjonali 18-19 ta' April 1991. Malta: Ministry of Education, 1991, 67-82; J. Viaud, 1981: op. cit.; E. Sykes, 1993: op. cit., 13,69,88-89; B. Brier: Egyptian Mummies. Unraveling the Secrets of an Ancient Art. M. London: O'Mara Books Ltd., 1996, 27; H.E. Sigerist, 1951: op. cit., 285-288

collection of apotropaic implements, and he was better equipped than anybody else to frighten away and chase off evil spirits and neutralize the evil eye. People therefore had him around whenever they felt particularly exposed to the spirits, and the parturient woman was considered to be at particular risk of falling prey to evil spirits because of her weakness and preoccupation. Bes thus presided over childbearing and was considered as a protector of expectant mothers. He was also a marriage-god and presided over the toilet of women. Toueris was another popular protective Egyptian goddess of childbirth, and symbolized maternity and suckling. She herself had given birth to the world. Toueris was represented as a female hippopotamus with pendant mammae standing upright on her back legs and holding the hieroglyphic sign of protection in one paw and the sign of life in the other. Amulets depicting the deity Ptah-Patecus have also been excavated. These depict the deity in his alternative form as a deformed dwarf with twisted legs, hands on hips and a huge head shaved except for the childish lock. Thus represented, Ptah plays the role of protector against noxious animals and against all kinds of evil. [26]

With the introduction of other religious cultures, the pantheon of protective deities was simply exchanged. With the advent of the monotheistic Christian religion in the fourth century ACE, the deities were replaced by venerated human individuals or saints. This led to the wearing of amulets depicting religious symbols such as the cross or images of saints. The use of amulets believed to have magical powers was also a frequent method used alone or as part of a magico-religious rite. These protective amulets also included papers containing decipherable or even indecipherable script sometimes containing extracts from the Gospels or the Koran. The reciting of prayers or "magical" incantations, sometimes read from a book, alone or associated with the laying of hands was also considered efficacious in the magical treatment of certain conditions. The practice was already prevalent during the

---

[26] J. Viaud: Egyptian Mythology. New Larousse Encyclopedia of Mythology. Hamlyn Publ, London, 1981, 9-48; H.E. Sigerist: A History of Medicine. Vol. I: Primitive and Archiac Medicine. Oxford University Press, New York, 1951, 241-242; C. Savona-Ventura: Outlines of Maltese Medical History. Malta, Midsea Publ., 1997, 8-9; C. Savona-Ventura: Punic Mythology and Medicine. Treasures of Malta, 2002, 8(3):83-88

32

sixteenth requiring Mgr Petrus Duzina during his 1575 Apostolic visit to enjoined priests to *"non si dice messa sopra l'hostie scritte carte, o`, orationi, o`, altre cose superstitiose, ne dia cosa alcuna sacra come cera, acquasanta, et simile cose a` laici, o` sospetti di superstitioni."* [27] In modern times the use of amulets in the form of crosses and images of saints is still prevalent, though these usually worn as accessory dress items rather than simply to protect against evil.

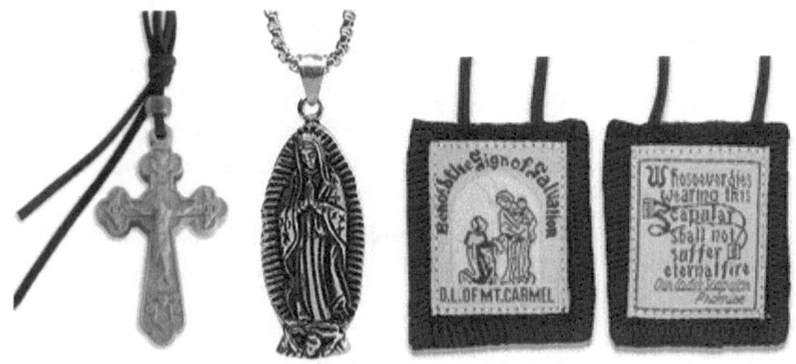

Modern Christian amulets
Cross – Our Lady – Carmelite scapular

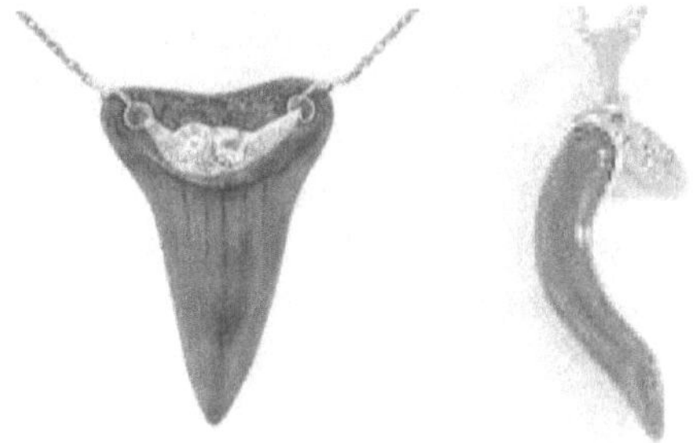

Modern Pagan amulets
Shark tooth - Horn

---

[27] G. Aquilina, S. Fiorini: Documentary Sources of Maltese History. Part IV Documents at the Vatican. No.1 Archivio Segreto Vaticano Congregazione Vescovi e Regolari Malta: Visita Apostolica no.51 Mgr. Petrus Dusina, 1575. University Press, Malta, 2001, f.381-381v

Witch-Doctor practices

When the protective measures fail and a breakdown in prehistoric man's vigilance to ward off evil occurs, then "internal" disease resulted. The treatment measures applied depended on the conceived cause and nature of the disease. Thus, if the cause was diagnosed to be religious, such as when a taboo was broken or actions which may incur the wrath of the spirits had been performed, then the ghost or deity needed to be appeased. If, on the other hand, the evil was the result of sorcery, then stronger magical powers would be required to overcome the illness. The medical practices of primitive man were thus closely intertwined with magico-religious rites and require the intervention of the medicine-man or shaman. The medicine-man in primitive societies was concerned not only with the people's health, but also with their entire welfare. It was his function to avert any evil which may threaten the individual or tribe in any form, to propitiate the spirits for the benefit of his people, and also to destroy the enemy. He was therefore priest, sorcerer and physician in one.[28]

There are strong indications that Late Neolithic man in Malta practiced shamanism, whereby priests or shamans had powers which could influence evil spirits which were the harbingers of disease and death. The administration of all healing procedures involves both visible (or audible) and invisible elements. Evidence of shamanism during the Temple Period was found at Brochtorff Circle in Gozo. Among the stone sculptured finds from the site was a cache of nine carved stone idols, associated with a miniature Tarxien Phase pot filled with ochre. The objects must originally have been wrapped tightly in a bag or box since they were all lying one above the other. Eight of the objects represent human figures, while the remaining idol has a pig's head. The context of the discovery suggests that these objects were the paraphernalia employed by shamans, probably in conjunction with the death cult.[29] The association of shamans or priests with the fertility cult can be evidenced by the definite sacrificial rituals which were carried out in the megalithic temples, while some of the portrait model statuettes excavated from various temple sites have been interpreted as representing temple

---

[28] Read, 1995, 256-274; Sigerist, 1967, 161-180

[29] Malone et al, 1995, 82

34

officials.[30] There can be no doubt that shamans were involved in the magical rituals associated with the fertility and death cults.

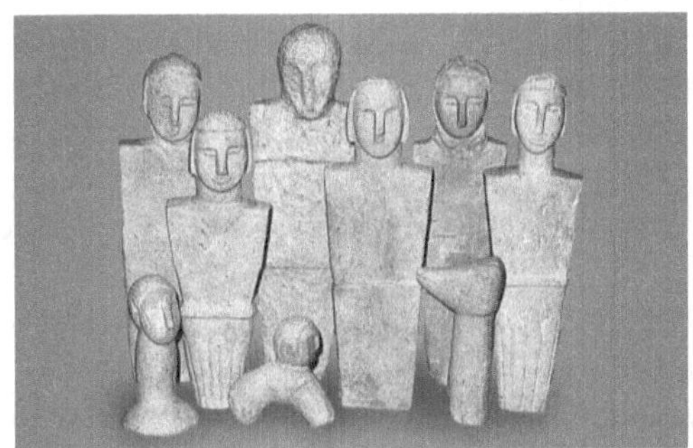

Shaman's tools used possibly during burial ritual – Xghara Circle

Furthermore, a number of statuettes interpreted as possible votive offerings have been excavated from Neolithic sanctuaries in Malta. Among these are two models of legs from Mnaidra, one of a hand from Hagar Qim, and a number of torso fragments from Hal Saflieni and Mnaidra. A limb from the Bugibba Temple showed a small conical knob on its lower part of the anterior aspect possibly representing a tumour. The feet of many of the obese statuettes are depicted as very short and plantiflexed suggestive of an artificial deformity, while some of the legs of statuettes found exhibit what may be marked oedema. A clay head shows puffed out cheeks possible representing angioneurotic oedema or bilateral parotitis, such as one get in mumps.[31]

The retrieval of the clay statuette suggestive of sympathetic magic rites and votive statuettes from various temple and hypogea sites may be interpreted to suggest that the medical shaman was the same as the temple and hypogea official. The shaman was probably also consulted in situations where disease was interpreted to be due to the invasion of the

---

[30] Zammit and Singer, 1924

[31] Zammit and Singer, 1924, 78,81,85,90-92,97-98; J.L. Pace. The anatomical features of prehistoric man in Malta. Malta: Royal University of Malta, 1972, 14; A.J. Agius. The Hal Saflieni Hypogeum. Malta: Union Press, 1968, 4-6; Zammit et al. 1912, 28

person by an evil spirit or ghost. In many prehistoric and even in primitive societies, this situation was remedied by embarking on trepanning of the skull to allow the evil spirit or ghost to leave the possessed.[32] Trepanation has not been described in Neolithic Maltese skulls. However, one of the skulls excavated from the Hal Saflieni Hypogeum in Malta (HS/2) shows an elliptical defect measuring about 15.5 x 12.7 mm on the left parietal bone, its medial edge being about 25.4 mm from the sagittal suture. The borders of this defect appear regular and are not likely to have been caused by accidental post-mortem trauma.[33]

On the basis of the two statuary remains depicting two women lying on a couch found at the Hal Saflieni Hypogeum, it has been suggested that this site served as a sanctuary in which "devotees were able to consult an oracle under the direction of a numerous priesthood who among other things practiced oneiromancy, that is they interpreted dreams provoked in the faithful that slept in cubicles". This practice is similar to the temple-hospitals of Asclepius of ancient Greece where, after acts of purification, the patient was brought to the holiest part of the sanctuary and instructed to lie down on a couch and await the coming of the god in a dream or vision, possibly brought on by the use of drugs. Thanks offerings in the form of votive offerings were then presented to the sanctuary.[34] There is however no definite proof that the practice of oneiromancy was prevalent in Late Neolithic Malta, and the statuary remains depicting sleeping women were probably related with the restful sleep of the death cult. The votive Neolithic objects excavated in Malta may be interpreted as ex-votos, offered as thanksgiving to the gods by sick devotees. A Classical Age temple dedicated to Asclepius is extant at Agrigento in Sicily. The Grecian deity Asclepius and his daughter Hygeia

---

[32] F.P. Lisowski. Prehistoric and Early Historic Trepanation. In D. Brothwell, A.T. Sandison (eds.). Disease in Antiquity. A survey of the Disease, Injuries and Surgery of Early Polulations. USA: C.C. Thomas, 1967, 651-672; E.L. Margetts. Trepanation of the skull by the Medicine-man of Primitive Cultures, with particular reference to present day Native East African Practice. In D. D. Brothwell, A.T. Sandison (eds.). Disease in Antiquity. A survey of the Disease, Injuries and Surgery of Early Polulations. USA: C.C. Thomas, 1967, 673-701

[33] Savona-Ventura and Mifsud, 1999

[34] Zammit and Singer, 1924; Cassar, 1964

36

was adopted in their pantheon of deities by the Romans and invoked in situations when illness prevailed.

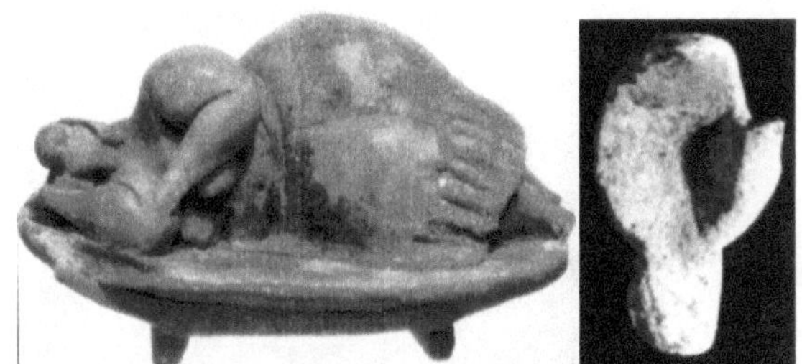

Possible votive offerings – Temple Period, Malta

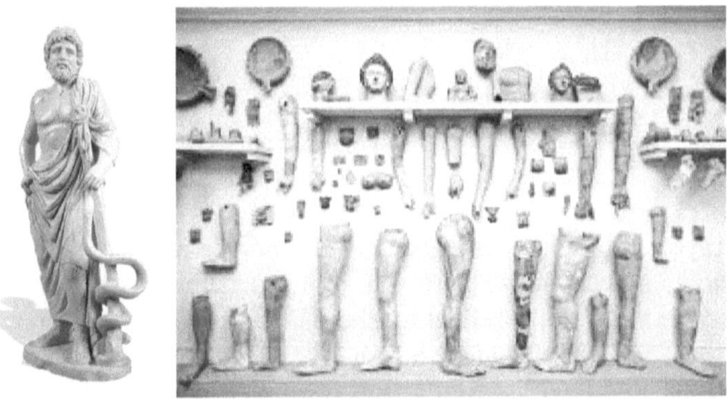

Votive offerings to Asclepius

The advent of Christianity brought a change in the concepts of pantheon of deities and the miraculous cures brought on by prayer and the 'laying of hands' described in the New Testament introduced these methods into the magico-religious management of illness. The first such incident practiced in Malta refers to the miraculous cure of the father of the Island's governor in 60 ACE from dysentery after the apostle Paul prayed and laid hands upon him.[35]

---

[35] Acts of the Apostles, 28:7-10, c.60 ACE

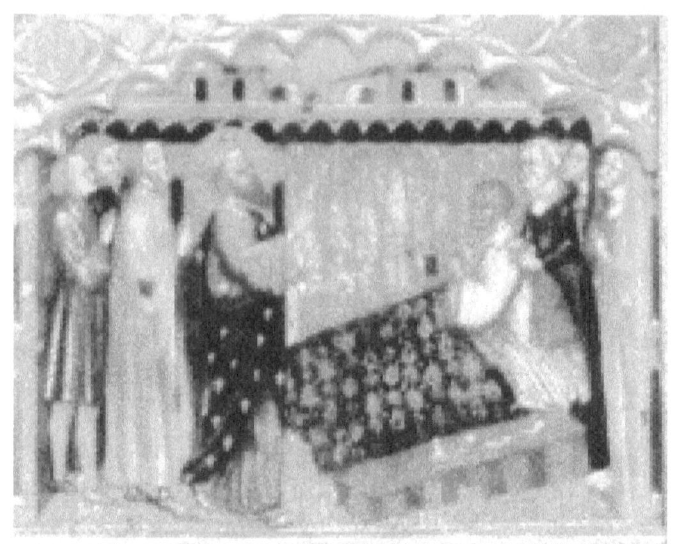

Apostle Paul healing sick from dysentery

Prayer and the laying of hands were universally adopted throughout the Christian world with particular powers being attributed to specific holy persons generally reflecting their hagiological story. Thus the 15th century ACE cave-chapel at St Agatha's Catacombs at Rabat and Hal Millieri at Siggiewi in Malta are decorated by a series of frescoes depicting several holy persons attributed with miraculous healing powers: St. Agatha – patron saint of breast disease; St. Blasé – protector of children with throat complaints; St. Lucy – patron saint of sight; and St. George – patron saint of skin disorders. There has also been the setting up after plague epidemics of a number of votive processions and dedicated chapels to patron saints associated with the infection: St. Sebastian, St. Basilius, St. Nicholas, and St. Roque.

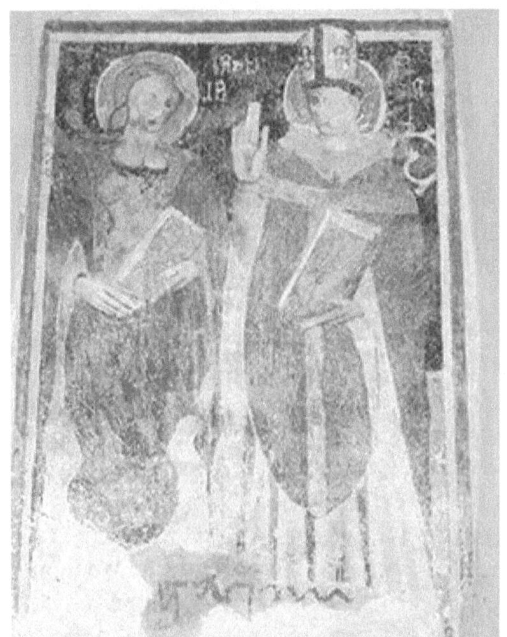

Frescoes at Hal Millieri Chapel, Malta
St. Agatha – St. Blaise

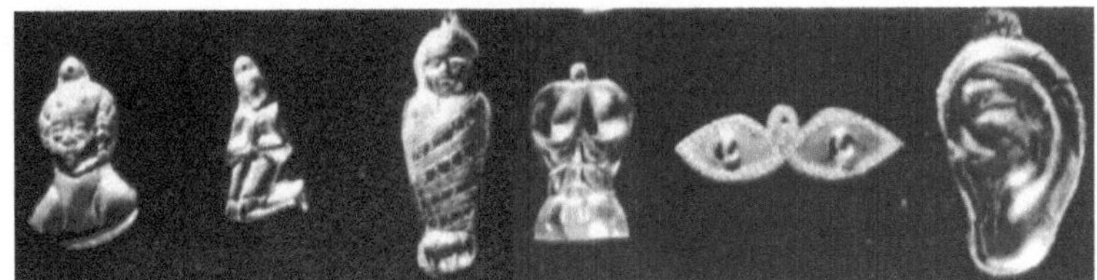

Votive offerings, Malta

Votive offerings were also deposited to bear witness to miraculous cures in places of worship generally dedicated to Mary, mother of Jesus – Shrines at Tal-Herba, Tal-Hlas, and Ta' Pinu churches. Votive offerings included ex-voto paintings depicting the disease or situation, e.g. a birth scene, and silver or wax models of the diseased organ or swaddled infant.[36]

While prayer and belief in the miraculous was generally promoted by the religious institution, the Roman Catholic Church set up a judicial court in efforts to combat superstitious beliefs especially when these verged on presumed witchcraft and alternative pagan beliefs. The Roman Inquisitional records in Malta suggest that during the seventeenth century no less than 28 percent of cases heard by Inquisitor Antonio Pignatelli dealt with sorcery resulting from folk religious practices with ten of the 64 cases being concerned with acts of healing. At the end of the eighteenth century, the number of cases concerning witchcraft had increased accounting for 37.8 percent of cases appearing before the tribunal.[37] These cases often combined a carrying mixture of folk and herbal medicine with semi-religious rituals.[38] The standard treatment in magico-religious rites was fumigation of the patient with burnt ingredients such as the smoke of a mixture consisting of oil blessed in honour of St. Peter the Martyr, a laurel leaf and a small piece of wood removed from the house door. Sometimes the burnt material included pieces of paper containing indecipherable writing. The rite used was occasionally even more complex. In 1631, a woman was advised fumigating the patient's head with fumes from the resin of the *Domema ammoniacum*. This was followed by mixing the ashes with water and using the mixture to make signs of the cross over the body joints. The remaining mixture was then to be thrown away while reciting an incantation. The rite of fumigation was occasionally closely linked to religious concepts. An elderly woman in 1789-1792 was treating jaundice patients by fumigation using a mixture of oil and candles blessed on the Day of Purification of Our Lady. During the fumigation she made the

---

[36] P. Cassar. Medical Votive Offerings in the Maltese Islands. The Journal of the Royal Anthropological Institute of Great Britain and Ireland, Jan-June 1964, 94(1):23-29

[37] C. Cassar. Witchcraft beliefs and social control in seventeenth century Malta. Journal of Mediterranean Studies, 1993, 3(2):331-334; A. Camenzuli. Maltese social and cultural values in perspectives - confessions, accusations and the Inquisitional Tribunal: 1771-1798. MA Thesis, University of Malta, 1999

[38] P. Cassar. Healing by sorcery in the 17th and 18th century Malta. St. Luke's hospital Gazette, 1976, 11(2):79-88

sign of the cross over the head, eyes and joints, and recited prayers to the Holy Trinity and Our Lady.

The belief that a person could be possessed by evil spirits was also prevalent. Possession was managed in various ways. In 1636, a woman whose illness was believed to have been due to bewitchment was told to bury one wax doll in her house and melt a second wax doll over a fire. This rite was believed to transfer the disease to the dolls, and by their destruction result in the destruction of the illness. One mother of a sick child in 1678 was told to bathe her child in water containing a particular herb while repeating three times the formula "Take your child and give me my own". Bathing was prescribed for various ailments. In 1636, a mother of sick child was similarly advised to wash the child with water containing the goose-foot plant ensuring that the no mention of the name of Jesus or the sign of the cross was made during the bathing. The belief of evil spirit possession is still prevalent in religious circles and members of the clergy are empowered to perform exorcism in such circumstances. In regular use during serious illness, the sacrament extreme unction is applied to give spiritual strength to the individual to combat the illness.

Conclusion

It would thus appear that medicine, mythology and religion probably all arose from the basic instinct for survival with the fertility and hunting cults being related to food procurement, while the dead cults and shamanism being related to ensuring good health. Ethnological parallels of the practices of prehistoric man in Malta with those of prehistoric man from other European regions and those of primitive communities suggest that in the face of common instincts and pressures, human responses tend to converge and are represented by common human responses aimed at satisfying basic supernatural needs.

Observational Medicine

Introduction

Traditionally, communities acquired a corpus of knowledge relevant to maintaining and restoring health that was passed down from one generation to the next. The corpus of knowledge related to healthy lifestyle advice, medical or surgical interventions, and herbal medicine.

Lifestyle interventions

The corpus of Maltese proverbs serves as a source of lifestyle interventions necessary for maintaining health including a correct dietary regimen and active way of life. [1] Proverbs are simple, concrete, traditional sayings that expresses a truth based on common sense or experience. They are often metaphorical and use formulaic language. Collectively, they form a genre of folklore that reflects the communal accumulation of knowledge throughout the ages. These cover a wide range of topics including interrelationships, family life, social betterment, prudence and good sense, and practical wisdom and foresight. Some relate to health living and lifestyle.

The Maltese have specific terms for gluttony often relating this to the nutritional habits of the pig. Thus, the word *"żaqqerija"* is entomologically derived from the Semitic word *"żaqq"* meaning "belly" and the Italian word *"porcheria"* meaning "nastiness" and "obscenity" itself derived from *"porco"* meaning "pig". *Żaqqerija* thus translates to "having the belly of a pig". Another related Maltese word meaning gluttony and greed is *ħneżrija* derived from the Semitic word *"ħanżir"* meaning "pig". The nutritional message in these proverbs is standard throughout – gluttony is harmful to one's health.

---

[1] J. Aquilina. A comparative dictionary of Maltese Proverbs. Malta: University Press, 1986

Min jibla' wisq imut qasir il-għomor.	He who eats too much dies young.
Bla ikel tmut, u l-ikel bosta jmewwet qasir il-għomor.	Without food one dies, too much food cuts life short.
Min m'għandux xaba' jifga.	He who is never sated will choke.
Iż-żaqq li ttiha tieħu.	The belly takes what you give it.
Aktar tmut in-bies bix-xaba' u le bil-ġuħ.	More people die from too much food than of hunger.
Iż-żaqqaktar ma tagħtiha aktar trid.	The more the belly gets, the more it wants
Għajnejh akbar minn żaqqu.	His eyes are bigger than his belly.
Imżaqq tajjeb isemmen.	Good food fattens.
Iż-żejjed (ħu in-)bħan-nieqes	Excess is similar (is brother) to deprivation.
Wara li tagħma, għalxejn tagħmel id-dieta	No use dieting after going blind

On the other hand, wellbeing is associated with good nourishment.

Ftit laħam isebbaħ qattus	A little flesh makes the cat lovely.
Il-qawwa, oħt il-ġmiel.	Good health [or stoutness] is the sister of beauty.
Is-simna sabiħa f'debba, aħseb f'xebba.	Stoutness makes a mare lovely let alone the maid.
Aħjar tħallas lill-furnar mit-tabib.	Better to pay the baker than the doctor.

The geographical characteristics of the Archipelago exposes the islands to an arid climate, absence of waterways and agricultural land restriction; factors that have resulted in the Islands being long dependant on food imports and having throughout history repeatedly been subject to periods of food restriction verging on starvation. Living in a restricted island environment with limited agricultural resources, the traditional Maltese diet was very rustic and dependent on the seasonal produce of the land and sea. Maltese cuisine has however been influenced by the interrelationship of the Maltese population with other circum-Mediterranean civilisations resulting in an eclectic mix of Mediterranean cooking being incorporated in the traditional Maltese cuisine. The lowered socio-economic status of the population throughout the centuries further contributed towards the population maintaining a frugal Mediterranean diet based on bread, vegetables, olive oil and fish. The

44

situation changed after the first quarter of the twentieth century when an increasing socio-economic status allowed the population to significantly alter its dietary habits to an Anglo-Italian one with an increase in the intake of animal fats and refined carbohydrates.[2] The long history of exposure to a restricted frugal Mediterranean diet led to epigenetic alterations to promote survival under low nutrition availability. This adaptive process drives the individual to become relatively insulin-resistant to promote towards higher level of circulating insulin and more efficient nutrient storage. The changes in nutritional habits, the insulin-resistant tendency has led to a greater predisposition of metabolic disease in the population with a high prevalence of obesity, type 2 diabetes mellitus, and hyperlipidaemia.[3]

An active working lifestyle was also considered positively with many proverbs promoting a long day of work.

Minn ibakkar fil-għodu jista' jorqod fil-għaxija	He who start work early in the morning can sleep during the night.
Bakkar u ishar [waħħar]	Get up early and keep on working till late.
Biex taqbad il-ħut trid tqum kmieni	To catch fish, one must get up betimes.
Il-bniedem l-inkwiet joqtlu mhux ix-xogħol.	Worry will kill man, not work.

However, the most relevant proverb relating to work and health is the one stating:

Ix-xogħol saħħa [balzmu][salmura tal-ġisem]	Work is health [balsam][bodily preserver].

---

[2] C. Cassar. Everyday life in Malta in the nineteenth and twentieth centuries. In: V. Mallia-Milanes, editor. The British Colonial Experience 1800-1964: The Impact on Maltese Society. Malta: Mireva Publ., 1988, 91-126

[3] C. Savona-Ventura & S. Savona-Ventura. Endogenous physiological teratogenesis – The Maltese population: A case-study. Germany: Lambert Academic Press, 2013

On the other hand, rest is essential to good heath:

L-irqad jagħmel il-ħmira.	Sleep makes the yeast [i.e. regenerates new energy]
Għix bil-mod u tgħix ħafna.	Live easily and you will live a long life.

A good mental outlook was also considered useful to wellbeing and excessive worrying served to no purpose:

Daħka bżonnjuża daqs ix-xemx.	A good laugh is as useful as the sun.
Mitt xejn qatel ħmar.	A hundred nothings killed an ass.
Il-marda li wieħed l-aktar jibża' minnha aktarx imut biha.	One generally dies of the illness one dreads most.
Aħjar is-saħħa mill-flus [mill-ġid kollu tad-dinja].	Better good health than money [all the wealth in the world]

Preventive measures to promote good health and prevent illness was also promoted.

L-indafa oħt il-qdusija [is-saħħa]	Cleanliness is sister to holiness [healthiness].
Il-mard trid tilqagħlu.	One must take preventive measures against illness.
Fejn tidħol ix-xemx ma jidħolx it-tabib.	Where the sun enters, the doctor does not.
Kulħadd tabib tiegħu nnifsu.	Everyone is his own doctor.
Saħħtek ibża għaliha; jekk ma hix fil-għana, faqar ma fiha.	Take care of your health; if it does not make you rich, it will not make you poor either.
Is-saħħa m'hemmx prezzha.	Good health is priceless.
Is-saħħa tkun taf kemm tiswa meta timrad [titlifha].	Health is appreciated when you get sick [loose it].

Other proverbs related to a healthy lifestyle and medical matters include:

Il-mard ikerrah u jbellah.	Disease makes one look ugly and foolish.
Sa l-erbgħin il-qabar miftuħ.	Till forty [days] the tomb is open [referring to risks of the puerperium to women].
Deni ta' kuljum fl-aħħar item.	Daily fever at last wears you away.
l-agħar l-ugħieħ tar-ras, tad-dras u l-ħlas.	The worst pains are headache, toothache, and labour pains.
Il-mard jidħol jigri u jmur bil-mod.	Sickness comes in quickly and goes out slowly.
Riħ tlitt ijiem biex jiġi, tlitt ijiem fis-sodda u tlitt ijiem biex imur.	A cold rakes three days to come, three days in bed, and three days to go.
Kull marid għandu d-duwa tiegħu.	Every sick person has his own medicine.
Ir-rigel trid is-sodda; u l-id il-maktur.	The bed for the leg and handkerchief for the hand.

Medical/Surgical interventions

The aetiology of traumatic lesions is immediately evident and thus not associated with a superstitious causation. Immediate remedies were implemented in these situations to stop active bleeding or splint fractures. Superficial lesions presenting at the skin similarly had an obvious causation and measures were undertaken to help relieve pain and release any pustular collections. These practical practices are evident in the "cures" promoted by Maltese medical folklore.[4]

In Maltese medical folklore, attempts at controlling bleeding from superficial lacerations was made using substances found at hand to promote coagulation. Items in popular use included the covering of the open wound with a spider's web, or the seeds of the Rock Phagnalon

---

[4] G.G. Lanfranco. Some recent communications on folk medicine in Malta. L-Imnara, 1980, 1(3):80-98; G. Lanfranco. Medicina populari ta' l-imghoddi fil-Gzejjer Maltin. Malta: Klabb Kotba Maltin, 2001

[*Phagnalon rupestre* - Maltese: *lixka*] or the Southern Cattail [*Typha domingensis* - Maltese: *buda*], or alternatively the fine downy feathers of the Grey Heron [*Ardea cinerea* - Maltese: *russet griz*]. Alternatively the wound was covered with powdered rice, ground limestone, or ground black pepper with the aims of promoting coagulation and sealing of the wound.

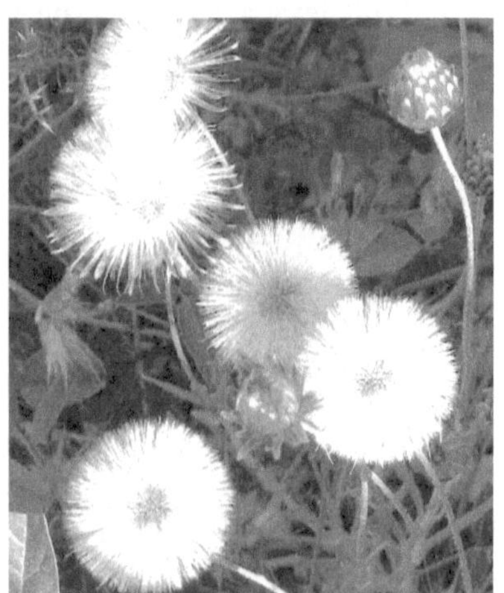
Rock Phagnalon

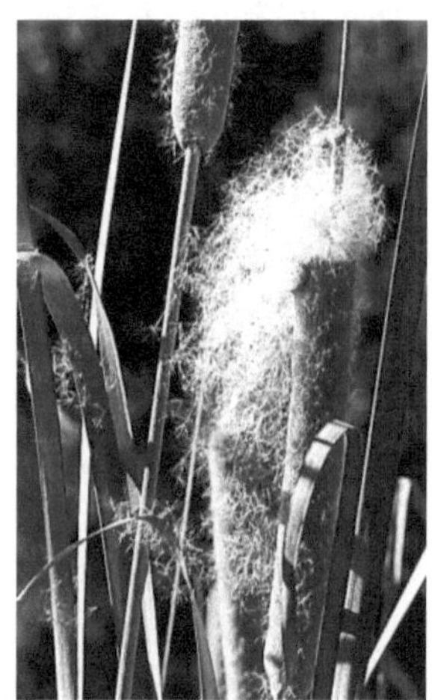
Southern Cattail

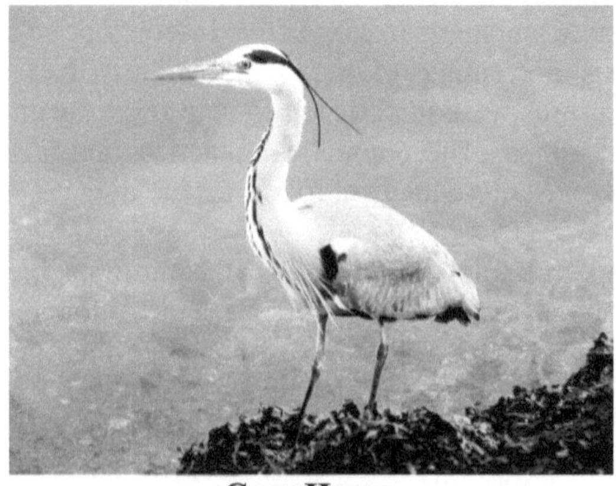
Grey Heron

Open wounds were dressed with sugar or honey, or alternatively covered with beaten egg-white. The use of eggs in the management of open wounds had a long usage in Malta dating to at least the mid-sixteenth century.[5] Before the discovery of microbes and antiseptics, infection and pus formation generally accompanied wound healing. The presence of pus – *'pus bonum et laudabile'* (good and laudable pus) – was generally considered a good sign indicative of eventual healing.[6] To promote suppuration, liquid ointments termed *unguenti digestivi* made from turpentine, basil, aloe tincture and egg-yolk were applied to open wounds. The use of this ointment has been recorded among the prescription list dated to 1546-47 being probably applied to open ulcers caused by venereal disease. In 1637, the Sardinian galley-surgeon Antonio Melin is known to have used egg-yolk to treat the wounded in battle. The Archives of the Order of Saint John for 1697-1706 further record that in July 1698, the surgeon at the *Sacra Infermeria* was being given a daily allowance of three eggs for the management of wounds. The preparation of *digestivi* involved triturating the egg-yolk or the egg-yolk and white with a fixed or volatile oil such as turpentine in a mortar while water was gradually incorporated. The resulting emulsion was finally strained to remove any strings of albumin. [7] The use of egg emulsion or honey for the management of open wounds continued well into the twentieth century.[8] The use of egg emulsion has now been replaced by hydrogel wound dressings, e.g. Gel-Syte ® or Intrasite Gel ®, that aim to create and maintain an optimal moist wound environment as this gently rehydrates sloughy and necrotic tissue which must be removed before healing can progress. They further absorb excess exudate, thereby halting the build-up of cellular debris and so help to prevent slough formation.

---

[5] C. Savona-Ventura. Eggs in the medical treatment of wounds. Sunday Times [Malta] 19th August 2001, p.18

[6] The rationale behind this was that the presence of pus suggested the presence of a staphylococcal infection rather than a streptococcal infection, the latter being more likely to spread throughout the tissues predisposing to septicemia.

[7] C. Savona-Ventura. Knight Hospitaller Medicine in Malta [1530-1798]. P.E.G. Ltd, Malta, 2004, p.193

[8] The author has himself seen senior gynaecologists manage the open wounds following a radical vulvectomy being managed with both egg emulsions and honey.

Similar use in the management of open wounds was the use of honey which because of its low pH, hyperosmolarity and the presence of oxidizing agents acts as a strong antibactericidal agent reducing the risk of infection in the wound.[8] Maggots were also used in the management of necrotic open wounds since these will feed only on dead flesh and leave behind a clean wound. The use of maggot therapy for wound debridement has been now re-adopted in surgical practice.[9]

Another reported method to dress open wounds was to prepare a specific oil-based balsam by beating an egg that had been laid on the 25th March [Feast day of the Annunciation] in oil. This mixture, after being left to stand, gave rise to an oil-based ointment known colloquially as the Balsam of the Annunciation *[Balzmu tal-Lunzjata]* which was thought to have miraculous properties and thus be useful in the management of open wounds and boils. Another ointment believed useful in managing infected wounds was one made from the extract in oil of the liver of the Gulper Shark [*Centrophorus granulosus* – Maltese: *zaghruna*].[10]

A number of plants products were also used in the management of different types of wounds. These included the leaves from the plants the Plantain [*Plantago sp.* – Maltese: *bizbula*], the Rue [*Ruta bracteosa* – Maltese: *fejgel*], the Monk's cowl [*Arum italicum* – Maltese: *garni*], and the Fox's Grapes [*Vitis labrusca* – Maltese: *gheneb id-dib*]. The latter was useful since the plant has further medicinal properties having substances with tranquillizer properties. The Rue plant was further used by boiling in oil and applying this to the open superficial wound. Similarly dried and powdered leaves of the Common Myrtle [*Myrtus communis* – Maltese: *rihan*] was used to dress open superficial skin wound. Leaves of the Sea ragwort [*Senecio cineraria* – Maltese: *Kromb il-bahar*] were bound on the open wound and the dressing changed frequently. The dried flowers and leaves of the Scurvy Pea [*Psoralea bituminosa* – Maltese: *silla salvagga*] were used on weeping wounds; while the General's Root

---

[9] C. Savona-Ventura. Invertebrates in the medical service of man: Part I – The Biotherapeutic Worms. Part II – The Insect Surgeons. Part III – The Research Assistants. The Synapse – The Medical Professional's Network, January 2007:14,18; March 2007:16-7; May 2007:16,28; February 2008: 12,20

[10] G.G. Lanfranco, 1980: op. cit.; G. Lanfranco, 2001: op. cit., 1-33

[*Cynomorium coccineum* – Maltese: *gherq il-general*] was used in haemorrhagic disorders and on open wounds. A poultice of the Common Elder leaves [*Sambucus nigra* – Maltese: *sambuka*] was used to manage ulcerations. [11]

The Wall Rue [*Ruta chalepensis* – Maltese: *fejgel*] or the leaves of the Borage [*Borago officinalis* – Maltese: *fidloqqom*] fried or seeped is oil was said to be useful to manage bruises. An alternative management was to rub the affected area with butter, while any swelling following a bump (a goose egg) could be managed by pressing a coin upon it. Leeching such bumps was not generally a method of choice. Alternatives to butter included a mix of Rue and oil or black or white ointment made from beeswax and oil. Other swellings were managed with Elder leaves decoctions [*Sambucus nigra* – Maltese: *Sebuqa Kbira, Sambuka*] generally placed in multiple of three [to represent the Holy Trinity – link to magico-religious beliefs]. For swelling in the ankle or feet, the limbs were to be soaked in an elder leaf water infusion. In the presence of inflammation, infusions of Rosemary or Barley were to be used. Alternatively a Bran poultice was also considered useful.[12]

Burn injuries were differently managed using substances whose primary aim was to refresh and cool the area. Items used in these situations included a tea infusion to serve as an astringent. A tea infusion was also used as a gargle in cases of a sore throat, as a mouthwash in cases of gingivitis, or as an eyewash in the presence of conjunctivitis. Alternative solutions used to manage burns included fresh milk, tepid bicarbonate solution, or urine. Various items were used to cover the burn. These included using a cataplasm made of the crushed leaves of the plant Coastal Stonecrop [*Sedum litoreum* – Maltese: *bezzul il-baqra*] or covered with the slit leaf of the Prickly Pear [*Opuntia ficus-indica* – Maltese: *bajtar tax-xewk*], or spreading a beaten egg white. Another burn covering option was the "silk" of the Noble Pen Shell [*Pinna nobilis* – Maltese: *nakkra tal-harir*]. Blisters were managed by applying a salt pack to help dry the lesion by the process of osmosis. Brine was also used to clean open wounds and also as a mouthwash in cases gingivitis. The

---

[11] G.G. Lanfranco, 1980: ibid; G. Lanfranco, 2001: ibid., 1-33
[12] G.G. Lanfranco, 1980: ibid; G. Lanfranco, 2001: ibid., 1-33

Vervan plant [*Verbena officinalis* – Maltese: *bukexrem*] was believed to be useful to manage carbucles and discolouration. It was also used in the management of fish stings. Rubbing the sting with warm urine or the liver of the poisonous fish such as the Scorpion fish [*Scorpaena scrofa* – Maltese: *skorfna*] or Spotted Weaver [*Trachinus radiatus* – Maltese: *tracna*] was also believed to be helpful. Chilblains could be managed by washing the hands in a warm infusion of Nettle [*Urtica membranacea* – Maltese: *Ħurrieq*]. [13]

The management of varicose veins involved the application of a poultice made of chamomile and bran, or mashed dry broad beans placed on the affected vein. Piles or haemorrhoids were managed by soaking these in an water infusion of maize fibre, garlic, or vinegar. Alternatively, one could sit over the vapour after boiling a mixture of garlic, chamomile and Pellitory [*Parietaria Judaica* – Maltese: *Xeħt ir-riħ komuni*] following which one went to bed. Alternative plants to use were Rough Bindweed [*Smilax aspera* – Maltese: *Zalza pajżana*], Garden Leek [*Allium ampeloprasum* – Maltese: *Tewm selvaġġ*], or Yarrow [*Achillea collina* – Maltese: *Ħaxixa tal-Morliti*]. For splenic problems, • boiled wall white land snails decoction were advocated. [14]

Various management options for pain from any aetiology were recommended. The primary basis of this management was the use of the principle of counter-stimulation, i.e. stimulating the painful region to reduce the pain sensation being caused by the injury or condition. This concept is based on the principles of the Gate and Humeral Theories of Pain. Thus for sprains or dislocations, the commonest remedy advocated was rubbing/massaging the painful part with a warm Rue infusion in oil. Alternative management options included rubbing the area with talcum powder, warm oil, or boiled thyme infusion. Poultices could also be used, especially in knee pain, using a hot poultice of mashed broad beans or bran and mustard powder. Pains of rheumatic origin could be managed using Squill bulb [*Urginea maritima* – Maltese: *Basal tal-għansar*], Cumin, or Rue applications. Sciatic pain was also said to be relieved by

---

[13] G.G. Lanfranco, 1980: ibid; G. Lanfranco, 2001: ibid., 1-33
[14] G.G. Lanfranco, 1980: ibid; G. Lanfranco, 2001: ibid., 1-33

rubbing the back with Squill or Rue. Alternatively, heat treatment using a warm brick wrapped in a cloth could be resorted to. Headaches were managed by placing sliced potato tubers or rubbing vinegar on the forehead. Toothache was managed by placing a clove nail or mustard near the offending tooth. An alternative was to dull the pain by placing some strong alcoholic beverage, e.g. whisky, on the tooth.[15] Earache could be managed by placing a cottonwool soaked in oil or the byssus fibres of the Pen Shell [*Pinna nobilis* – Maltese: *Nakkra*] while tying a handkerchief around the head to keep the ears warm. The management of excessive earwax included a procedure involving placing a paper cone into the ear canal and burning this to about half way before putting out the flame.[16] Presumably the warmth helped melt the wax allowing it to drain out. Inflammation of the eyes was managed by washing with a cold tea or camomile infusions. [17]

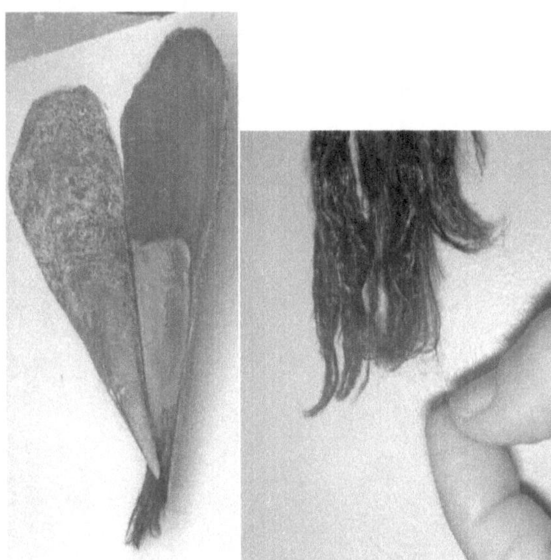

Pen Shell with byssus fibres

---

[15] G.G. Lanfranco, 1980: ibid; G. Lanfranco, 2001: ibid., 1-33
[16] This earwax management is also common in Sicilian traditional medicine.
[17] G.G. Lanfranco, 1980: ibid; G. Lanfranco, 2001: ibid., 1-33

A form of using counter-therapeutic principles was employed in the management of fever. The recommendation was that in the presence of fever, a rabbit was cut open and placed on the patient's abdomen. When the rabbit's tissue darkened or developed a smell, then the patient's fever would have been taken up by the carcass and the patient cured. Alternatively, a puppy could also be used instead of a rabbit. Other suggested remedies for feverish conditions consisted of drinking donkey's milk, placing a sliced potato onto the forehead leaving it there until it darkened. A poultice of boiled flax placed on the patient's back or chest was also advocated. Venesection or leeching was also used to reduce the inflammatory process. Other measures to manage fever was to rub oil or place oil mixed with baker's yeast on the palms and/or soles of the feet to draw out the fever. [18]

---

[18] G.G. Lanfranco, 1980: ibid; G. Lanfranco, 2001: ibid., 1-33

Rationalization of Medicine

Magico-religious rationalization

Man has always tried to identify a rational cause for important life events. The first attempt at rationalization led to the association of illness to religion and the occult. Thus, an acute-onset illness was perceived as a punishment from the contemporary deities for misdemeanours by the individual or the community. This would particularly account for epidemic disease affecting a large proportion of the community or alternatively a particularly bad harvest resulting in famine. Alternatively, an acute-onset disease in an individual would have been interpreted as a "magic shot" where something evil (such as an evil spirit or magical intervention) would have "entered" the individual. A chronic debilitating disease state would have been perceived as a loss of a vital essence extracted from the individual by a deity or through magical intervention.

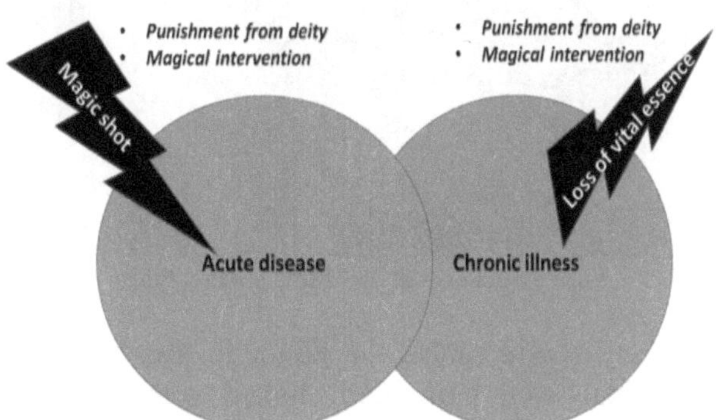

Magico-religious rationalization of disease

Such beliefs have persisted throughout the ages even when a other alternate explanations were prevalent. To a certain extent, it still plays a role in modern times. Acutely sick individuals often resort to supplement their medical management by resorting to prayers. Evidence for this practice can be seen by the deposition of votives evidence in many churches on the island. This reliance of the supernatural in itself may have a beneficial effect on the individual's facilitation of personal growth and psychological resilience in dealing with one's health challenges.[19] In the Roman Catholic culture, this spiritual assistance is formally administered through the sacrament of Extreme Unction or Anointing of the Sick. This is administered to any Catholic who, having reached the age of reason, begins to be in danger due to sickness or old age. The sacrament is administered by a priest, who uses olive oil or another pure plant oil to anoint the patient's forehead and perhaps other parts of the body while reciting certain prayers. It is believed to give comfort, peace, courage and, if the sick person is unable to make a confession, even forgiveness of sins.

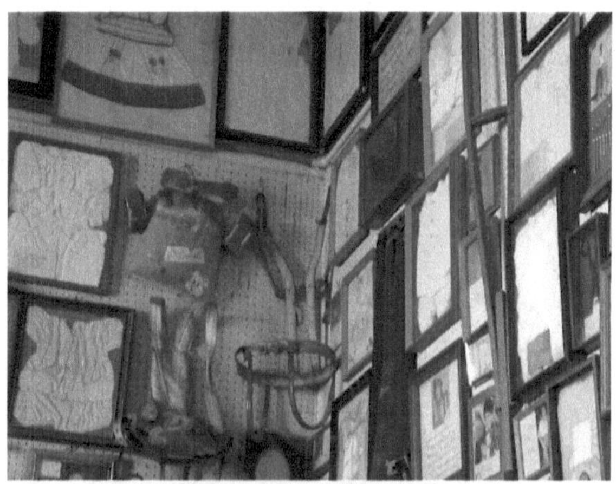
Votive offerings at Ta' Pinu Shrine, Gozo

Up to relatively recent times, the belief in the "evil eye" was still prevalent. Individuals were particularly linked to the power of inflicting the "evil eye" on individuals or object causing ill-health or damage. Amulets, including cowrie seashells or fragments of the red candles used before Good Friday, were worn as protection.[20] When perceived as

[19] D.M. Steinhorn, J. Din, A. Johnson. Healing, spirituality and integrative medicine. Ann Palliat Med. 2017 Jul;6(3):237-247
[20] G. Lanfranco. Medicina populari ta' l-imghoddi fil-Gzejjer Maltin. Malta: Klabb Kotba Maltin, 2001, 166

threatened by the "evil eye", protective measures were made by making the sign of the *Qrun* (direct translation is a bull's horn) by pointing outwards the index and little fingers.[21] In addition, it was believed that putting a line of salt on the floor behind the front door will prevent the evil eye from entering your house; while if one believed that the home had negative energies, then this could be cleansed by burning olive tree leaves at midnight on Easter while saying prayers (*Tbahhir*). There was also the belief that anyone could "magically" curse you should they acquire something personal. To prevent such occasions when personal items may be made available [e.g. after a haircut], then spitting on your hair before throwing it away was an option.

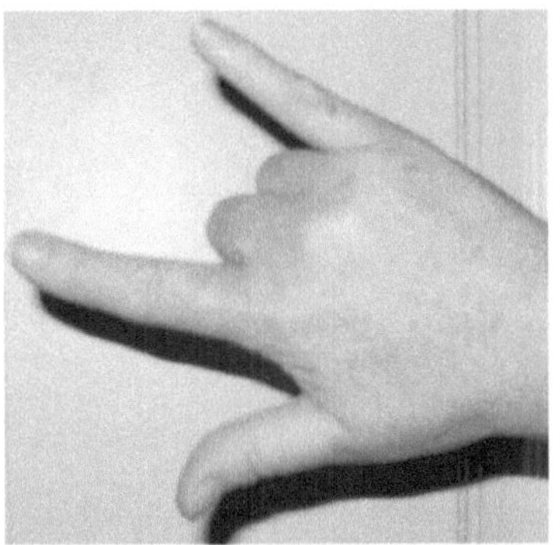

The Qrun to protect against the evil eye

Philosophical rationalization

The move to rationalize medical observations separating these from the magico-superstitious is attributed to the Greek physician Hippocrates. Hippocrates of Kos (~460—~370 BCE) was a Greek physician who revolutionized medicine in ancient Greece, establishing it as a profession. He is credited with coining the Hippocratic Oath of medical practice ethics, still relevant today. His school is credited with the introduction of the systematic study of clinical medicine, and the summing up the

---

[21] G. Zammit Maempel. The Evil Eye and protective cattle horns in Malta. Folklore 1968, 79:1-16

medical knowledge of the time. The systematic rational approach to medicine was integrated with the Ancient Greece concepts of the four elements – earth, water, air, and fire – which supposedly explained the nature and complexity of all matter. This led to the development of the Galenic Theory of the four humours and the rational belief that imbalance in the humours resulted in ill-health (Galen of Pergamum 129-219 ACE).

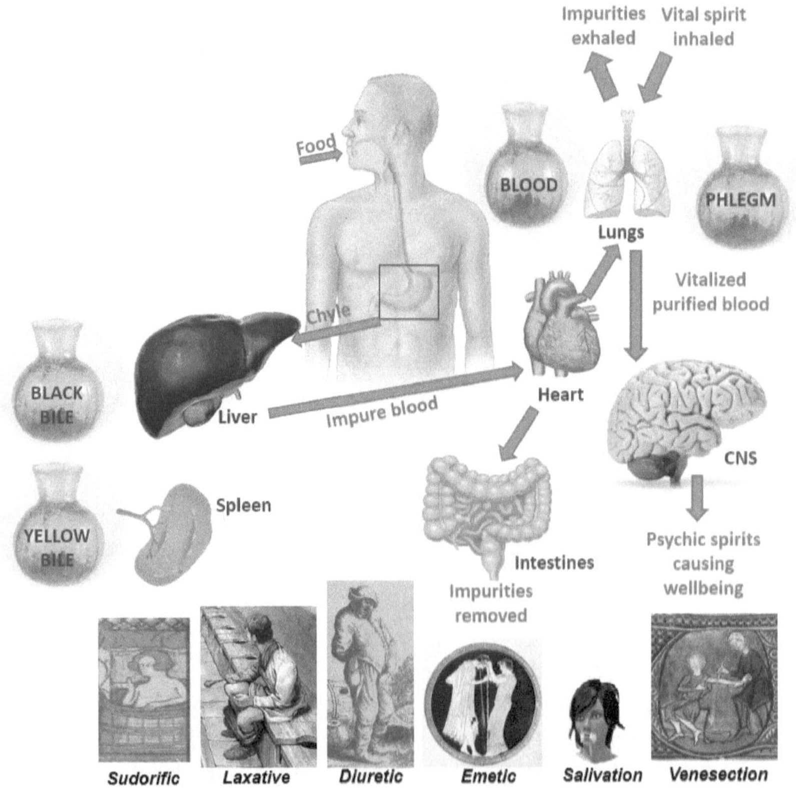

Galenic Theory of the Four Humours

Since ill-health was perceived to be the result of an imbalance of these four basic humours, therapeutic measures were developed in order to restore the balance. These measures centred on the use of laxatives,

58

emetics, diuretics, sialagogues to increase salivation, sudorifics, and venesection.

During the Early Modern Period, the Galenic principles were further extended to further rationalize the personalities exhibited by different individuals – the phlegmatic prone to apathy, the sanguine prone to optimism, the melancholic prone to sadness, and the choleric prone to anger.

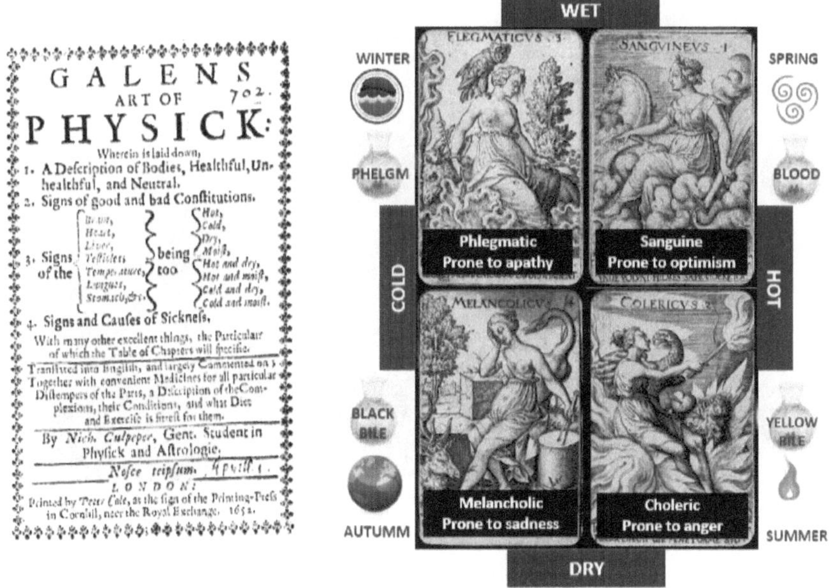

Galenic theory explaining personality

The first evidence of the adoption of the Galenic theory in the Maltese Islands dates to the Roman Period. A *Collegia funeratica* tomb slab at the necropolis sited outside the capital city of the island of Malta in use during the period 300-800 ACE shows a series of surgical instruments that include two bleeding cups used to facilitate venesection. The tomb slab served the purpose of sealing up one of the tombs in the catacomb complex.[22] Similar-shaped cups have been depicted on other tomb slabs and found in various archaeological sites in Europe. The practice of cupping [*fintusi* in the Maltese vernacular] with or without associated venesection remained an integral part of Maltese traditional practice rights up to the twentieth century.

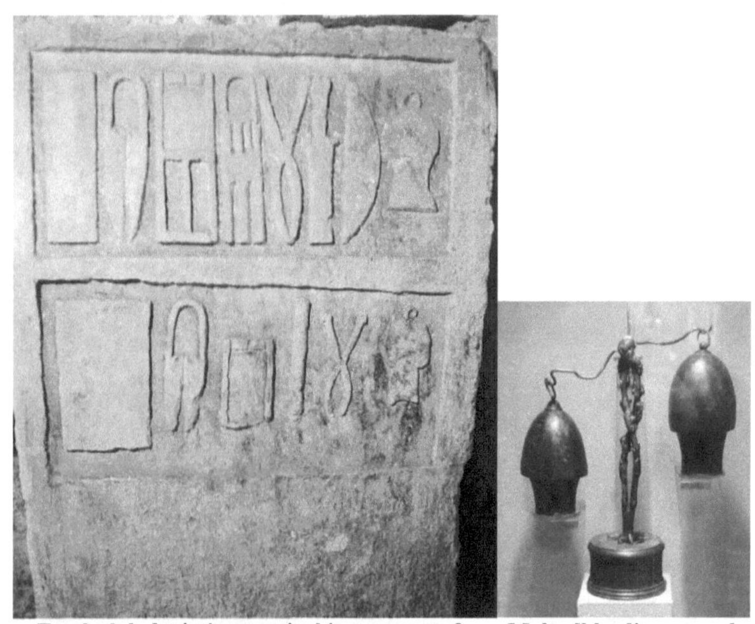

Tomb slab depicting surgical instruments from Malta [bleeding cups shown one above the other on the right] and 2nd century cupping kit excavated from doctor's grave at Bingen am Rhein in Germany.

Cupping, combined with venesection, became the mainstay management to restore health equilibrium during the Classical Period through the Middle Ages right to the 18th century. Cupping or the application of *fintusi* involved the application of vacuumed glass cups in specific regions over the body, usually but not restricted to the back. In traditional Maltese practice, cupping was generally used to alleviate

---

[22] P. Cassar. Surgical instruments on a tomb slab in Roman Malta. Medical History, 1974, 18:89-93

60

muscular pains, lumbago and sciatica, fever, mental disease and for a number of other non-specific illnesses. The methodology in general use in Malta involved a heat source which was usually a small piece of cloth lightly soaked in spirit or a small piece of candle placed on coin. After setting up and lighting the heat source, a cup in the form of a normal table tumble or a specifically designed cup was applied over the heat source. The burning process removed the oxygen contained in the cup extinguishing the heat source and causing a vacuum effect.[23] The mechanism of action of cupping, especially in regard to the relief of pain, is difficult to explain but may be assumed to work by acting as a method of counter-stimulation based on distraction in one location with the goal of lessening discomfort and/or inflammation in another.

Cupping has a long tradition of use in medical therapeutics. Counter-stimulation in the form of cupping during the prehistoric period was also prevalent in Ancient Egypt. The Ebers Papyrus dated to about 3550 BP refers to cupping for removing foreign noxious matter from the body. Archaeological depictions of cupping utensils have been described in the ancient medical instruments drawing on the wall of the temple Kom Ombo in Egypt.[24] The practice remained widespread throughout the Mediterranean region in the subsequent centuries.[25] Evidence of the possible use of counter-irritation to treat disease states in prehistoric Maltese tradition may include a small baked clay statuette depicting a naked pregnant female form excavated from the Tarxien Neolithic Temples. This statuette has a number of white shell fragments stuck into it when it was still wet and obviously purposefully impacted within the clay before firing in various parts of the body. These fragments are found in the neck, in the umbilicus, on the mons veneris, in both groins, in the base of the figure, on two of the ribs, three of the vertebra and on both scapulae.[26] It can be suggested that this model actually indicates pressure points where counter-stimulation may be applied in a pregnancy

---

[23] G.G. Lanfranco, 2001: op. cit., 125

[24] C. Savona-Ventura. Ancient Egyptian Medicine. Lulu, U.S.A., 2017, 21

[25] P. Mehta, V. Dhapte. Cupping therapy: A prudent remedy for a plethora of medical ailments. J Tradit Complement Med. 2015 Jul; 5(3): 127–134.

[26] Zammit and Singer, 1924, 96-97; Cassar, 1964, 4

condition/s.[27] The various bone implements excavated from various Temple Period sites in Malta may themselves have been also used to supplement the counter-stimulation procedure. These are similar to the sharp-ended bone needles and bian blades unearthed from the Neolithic archaeological sites in China. The small earthenware cup excavated from The small earthenware cup measuring 7.3 cm high excavated from Hal Saflieni Hypogeum may have possibly been used as a cupping vessel.[28]

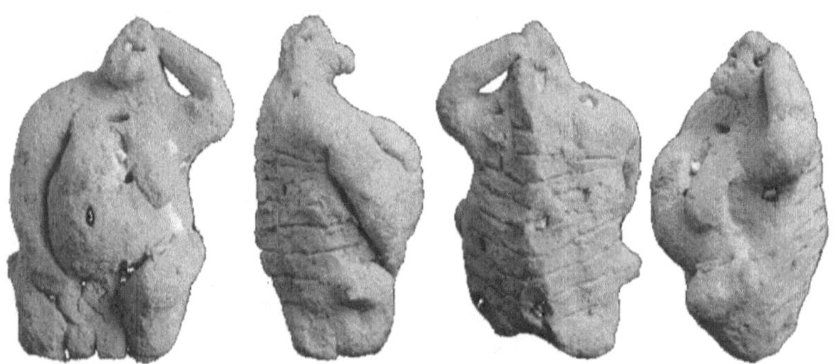

Pregnancy statuette from Tarxien Temple complex showing impacted shell fragments – witchcraft or counter-irritation pressure points

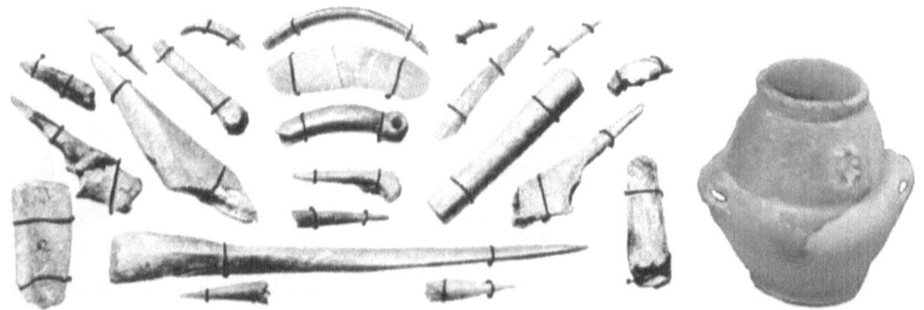

Bone implements including needles and earthenware cup excavated from Temple Period sites in Malta

---

[27] P. Cassar. Medical history of Malta. Wellcome historical Medical library, London, 1965, 4

[28] J.D. Evans. The Prehistoric antiquities of the Maltese Islands. University of London: London; 1971, p.62.

A method of counter-stimulation used in traditional Maltese medicine was the application of cataplasms, poultices and sinapisms. These substances were supposed to cause irritation or mild inflammation where applied and thus act as a counterirritant. A medical dressing made of a soft heated mass of meal or clay was spread on a cloth and applied to the skin to treat inflamed areas or improve the circulation at the site and manage local pain. They were also used to decrease swelling. The dressing was potentially made out of clay, linseed flour, bread, yeast or mustard. Charcoal was occasionally added with dressing made using clay, linseed flour or bread.[29] The first list of pharmacological agents mentioned in the historical record in Malta dates to 1345 when these items had a 10 percent tax imposed upon their importation. The 19 products listed in the *Capitula Sagati* of 1345 included mainly items of botanical origin but included *bolu* (medicinal clay) imported for medicinal use.[30] A series of prescriptions of the 16th century clearly demonstrates the use of the various therapeutic options to attempt cure disease by balancing the humours. A case of trauma had a cataplasm of *quinque farinarum* applied, while he further had two lotions of *fusco* and *Aegypciaco* applied to his wounds. He also received oil and honeyed extracts of oil of roses that were attributed with sedative properties. A second case involving trauma was prescribed an *unguenti digestive* made from turpentine, basil, aloe, tincture and eggs applied to an open wound.[31] cataplasms, poultices and sinapisms continued to be used in medical practice right up to the 20th century with specific instructions about their preparation being gives to nursing students in 1904.[32]

Various types of poultices were also used to help mature abscess formation. A number of these were used in traditional Maltese medical practice. These served their purposes either by the direct application of heated materials or by the materials themselves generating heat. In addition, some materials would have served as an emollient helping to

---

[29] S. Galizia. Il Ctieb ta l'Infermier. Lezionijiet mghotia lil infermieri ta li Sptar. Government Printing press, Malta, 1904, 84-100

[30] S. Fiorini. Kura u Servizzi tas-Sahha f'Malta sa nofs is-seklu XVI. In: Oqsma tal-kultura Maltija (T. Cortis, ed.) Ministry of Education, Malta, 1991, 233-234

[31] S. Fiorini. A prescription list of 1546. Maltese Medical Journal, 1988/89, 1(1):19-31

[32] S. Galizia, 1904: op. cit.,

soften the skin overlying the abscess allowing this to point and eventually drain. To help a boil to point, poultice made out of boiled leaves of the Butcher's broom plant [*Ruscus aculeatus*], mashed pumpkin [*Cucurbita pepo* – Maltese: *qara hamra*], long marrow leaves [Maltese: *qara twila*], simply bread crumbs and milk were often advocated, or an ointment made from almond oil mixed with sugar were advocated. Other useful options to help manage boils included the leaves of Mallow [*Malva sylvestris.* – Maltese: Ħobbejża tar-raba], Fennel [*Foeniculum vulgare* – Maltese: *Buzbiez*], or Walnut [*Juglans regia* – Maltese: *gellewza*]. Less significant skin infections such as eczema were treated using a oil-based decoction of wild thyme flowers [*Thymus capitatus* – Maltese: *saghtar*], or Kohlrabi tulip leaves [*Brassica oleracea* – Maltese: *gidra*].[33]

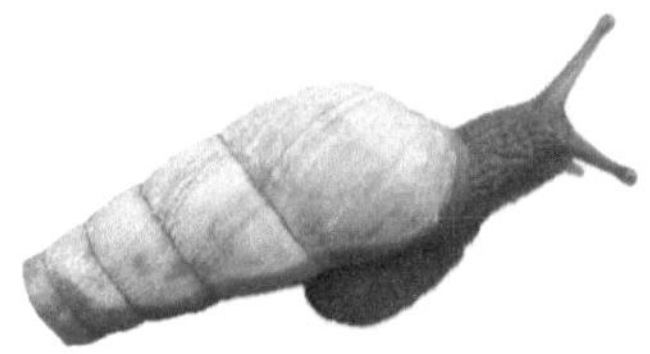

Decollate snail

Foot abscesses were similarly managed but other forms of treatment advocated included bandaging overnight a roasted onion over the lesion or the application of a oil-based poultice made from a ground land Decollate snails [*Bulimus decollatus*]. Whitlows were similarly managed, though another recommended management was to insert the affected finger in boiling water or alternatively warm the finger with a cloth dripped in boiling water. Foreign bodies were also similarly managed. The advocated management for sea urchin spines was to primarily attempt their extraction but, if unsuccessful, they were managed by bandaging overnight a roasted onion over the area. Other poultices were used as emollients aimed at softening hardened skin conditions like corns. These natural emollients included repeatedly applying overnight slices of

---

[33] G.G. Lanfranco. Some recent communications on folk medicine in Malta. L-Imnara, 1980, 1(3):80-98

the prickly pear leaves or tomato, or simply bread crumbs soaked in vinegar. [34]

Venesection remained an important management option in a large variety of disease right up to the beginning of the 20th century being carried out by direct lancing of a vein, or by using scarificators that made multiple incisions on the skin to cause multiple bleeding points, or by the application of leeches.[35] Venesection in small repeated quantities was regularly used in the management of fevers; while in the presence of wounds, the procedure was believed to reduce the inflammatory reaction by helping the absorption of extravasated blood from the tissues. The procedure was also used to prevent the development of pregnancy eclampsia, cerebral stroke, and in the management of severe headache, pulmonary oedema, mental disease and gastric symptomatology. Venesection was generally performed on the jugular or brachial veins, rarely from the veins of the leg. It was sometimes combined with cupping to help extract a larger volume of blood. Leeches were also applied to reduce superficial inflammation at wound sites especially after plastic surgery such as rhinoplasty.[36] This concept has been re-adopted in modern medicine using the anticoagulant injected by the leech to help with improving the circulation after plastic surgery.[37]

The practice of venesection in Malta persisted through the ages. In 1539, the procedure was being carried out by the barber-surgeons against payment of one *unza*.[38] A prescription of the 16th century clearly demonstrates the use of the various therapeutic options to attempt cure

---

[34] G.G. Lanfranco, 1980: idid.

[35] C. Savona-Ventura, R.T. Sawyer, P.J. Schembri. The Medicinal Use of Leeches in Malta. Malta Medical Journal 2002 14(1):48-52

[36] C. Savona-Ventura. Contemporary Medicine in Malta [1798-1979]. P.E.G. Ltd, Malta, 2004, 471-479

[37] C. Savona-Ventura. Invertebrates in the medical service of man: Part I – The Biotherapeutic Worms. Part II – The Insect Surgeons. Part III – The Research Assistants. The Synapse – The Medical Professional's Network, January 2007:14,18; March 2007:16-17; May 2007:16,28; February 2008: 12,20

[38] S. Fiorini. The Mandati' Documents at the Archives of the Mdina Cathedral, Malta 1473-1539. Minnesota: Hill Monastic Manuscript Library, 1992, xxii

disease by balancing the humours. A teenage child suffering from kidney problems received a "constrictive cataplasm ….. to harden and warm … the kidneys". He was also prescribed *pillule foetidae* and *opopanax* to evacuate "the cold rather crude and even bilious mood". Further prescriptions in the form of *pillulae aggregativae* were also prescribed to aggregate the humours prior to dispelling them with the assistance of the prescription *Jera pigra Galieni* which was supposed to "purge the stomach and cleanse the blood".[39] A 1542 medico-legal certificate from the Maltese ecclesiastical court confirms that the local medical practitioners – Giuseppe Callus and Rayneri Bonellis – were familiar with the medical works of authors supporting the Galenic Theory including Galen (c.131-200), Rhazes (860-932), Avicenna (980-1037), and Avenzoar (1072-1162).[40]

Venesection in small repeated quantities was regularly used in the management of fevers. In the management of wounds, the procedure was believed to reduce the inflammatory reaction to wounds by promoting the absorption of extravasated blood from the tissues. The quantity of blood removed depended on the constitution and temperament of the patient; with the "*sanguine*" individual being bleed freely while the "*bilious*" individual only sparingly. Bleeding was contra-indicated in the "*melancholic*" individual. The jugular and brachial views where most often used, but leg veins were occasionally resorted to. [41]

The gentler form of bloodletting through the use of leeches was also practiced in Malta. The first traced reference to the use of leeches in relation to the Maltese Islands dates to the late 16th century. Dr. Pietro Parisi from Trapani in Sicily, sent to Malta by the Viceroy of Sicily, left a detailed eyewitness description of the events that occurred during the Plague epidemic that ravaged the Maltese Islands during 1592-93. In his account, Parisi described the prevalent treatment for the disease, treatment that had

---

[39] S. Fiorini. A prescription list of 1546. Maltese Medical Journal, 1988/89, 1(1):19-31

[40] P. Cassar. A Medico-legal report of the sixteenth century from Malta. Medical History, 1974, 18:354-359

[41] M.A. Grima. Della medicina traumatica altrimenti detta vulneraria. Firenze, 1773, 45

undergone no change since the medieval period. Bloodletting was carried out in cases of plague in the belief that the procedure relieved the body of its noxious humours. Parisi advocated the use of leeches in conjunction with venesection, allowing the latter procedure to be dispensed with in timid patients, such as women and children, stating that "At times over the site of phlebotomy were placed three, or four leeches; so that they could suck out that virulent blood. And this should be performed on children & women because of their timidness, & not to feel the pain of the lancet, in such instances one may apply the said leeches without the primary venesection, once these detach themselves it is necessary to wash the site with tepid water, to ensure that no immediate ailment occurs to the bites, & allow the blood to ooze".[42]

The specific use in 1686 of leeches or "*Sanguisughe*" is recorded in a seventeenth century pharmaceutical register which lists the medicaments supplied to individuals belonging to the Order of Jesuits resident in the capital city of Malta during the period 1683-1713.[43] The medical application of leeches, in addition to venesection and cupping, is also recorded in the '*Commissari degli spogli*' applications of the mid-eighteenth century. Any creditors of a deceased Knight of the Order of St. John were obliged to apply for their dues to the Order's '*Commissari degli spogli*' to be remunerated from the knight's effects or '*spogli*' at the time of his death.[44] The leeches were generally applied by the barber-surgeon. The 1725 regulations of the main hospital in Malta, the *Sacra Infermeria*, define the duties of the barber-surgeon or phlebotomist to include the use of leeches.[45] Leeches applied to the temple have also been recorded in the eighteenth century as useful to prevent or reduce the inflammatory reaction that occurred in the eyeball

---

[42] P. Parisi. Avvertimenti spora la pesta e febre pestifera con la somma delle loro prencipali cagioni. Palermo: G.A. de Franceschi, 1593, 164-165,190.

[43] P. Cassar. Two centuries of medical prescribing in Malta 1683-1882. St. Luke's Hospital Gazette, 1969, 4(2):105-112

[44] P. Cassar. A note on the economics of medical practice in eighteenth century Malta. St. Luke's Hospital Gazette 1974b, 9(2):166-172

[45] Notizia della Sacra Infermeria e della carica delli Commissarj delle Povere Inferme. Rome: R. Bernaba, 1725 [English translation: E.E. Hume. Medical Work of the Knights Hospitallers of Saint John of Jerusalem. Baltimore: J. Hopkins Press, 1940, 137-148]

following firearm injuries to the orbital region [46]. In cases of headache and mental disorders, A slave-healer, prescribed venesection together with the application of ice on the head and hot baths to the feet.[47]

The danger of repeated venesection in causing anaemia was referred to by Dr. F. Butigiec in 1804 when he condemned the routine bloodletting to which pregnant women resorted to during the seventh month of pregnancy, this being performed in part as a precautionary measure against the development of eclampsia.[48]   The schedule of fees published in 1821 specifically refers to procedures such as applying a blister [fee: 1 *scudo* 3 *tari*], venesection, cupping or the application of leeches [fee: 6 *tari*], urethral catheterization [fee: 2 *scudi* 6 *tari*]; reduction of a hernia [fee: 3 *scudi*]; and operation for dropsy [fee: 2 *scudi* 6 *tari*]. Other surgical procedure such as the dressing of wounds, treatment of fractures, amputations, etc. were charged according to circumstances and time employed after submission to the Medical Committee.[49]

In 1816, the British physician W. Burnett, practicing in the British Naval Mediterranean Station, described the employment of leeches when less profuse bleeding was required in the treatment of cases of Mediterranean fever. From three to twelve leeches were applied to the temples in cases of severe headache, or to the epigastric region when gastric symptoms became troublesome. To ensure a continuous flow of blood, a cupping glass was applied over the orifices made by the leeches. In this way up to twelve ounces of blood could be procured.[50] Medical practitioners working in Malta similarly reported their use of leeches in specific medical

---

[46] M.A. Grima 1773: op. cit., 57

[47] P. Cassar. Healing by Sorcery in 17th and 18th century Malta. St. Luke's Hospital Gazette 1976b, 11(2):79-88

[48] F. Butigiec. Trattato dell'Arte Ostetrica dettato e spiegato dal Perille Signo Dr. Francesco Butigiec nello Studio Publico del Grand Ospedale de' Maltesi. Principiato li 18 Ottobre 1804. Manuscript lecture notes, +247f

[49] Minute by His Honor the Lieutanant Governor. Malta Government Gazette [MGG], 28th March 1821, 387:2567-2568. Currency conversion: 10,000 scudi were equivalent to about £stg 833; 12 tari equaled 1 scudo equivalent to about 1s8d.

[50] W. Burnett. Practical account of the Mediterranean Fever as it appeared in the Ships and Hospitals of His Majesty's Fleet in that Station during the years 1808, 1811 and 1813 and of the Gibraltar and Carthagena Fever. London: Callow, 1816

conditions. When the invalid Sir Walter Scott reached Malta in 1831, he exhibited symptoms of an impending stroke. He was attended by Dr. John Davy, then a military doctor stationed in Malta, who prescribed the application of leeches to Scott's head.[51]

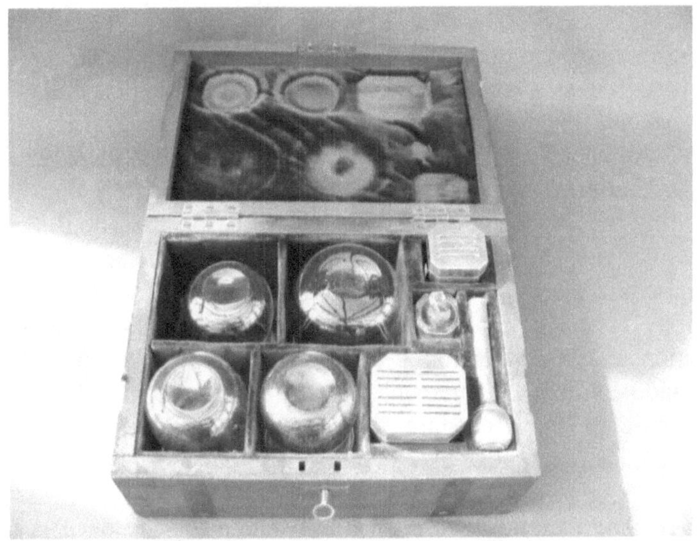

19ᵗʰ century cupping set with scarificator

Venesection was also a therapeutic option in the management of psychotic disease in an attempt to calm the excited individual. In Malta, venesection using lancing and leeches for psychotic conditions was advocated by Dr. T. Chetcuti in 1838.[52] Another method of venesection, considered more merciful than the other blood-letting instruments, in vogue during the 18ᵗʰ century was through the use of the scarificator. This device, containing a series of twelve blades, was cocked and the trigger released spring-driven rotary blades which caused many shallow cuts.

---

[51] P. Cassar. Physiological and Pathological Research at the General Military Hospital of Valletta, Malta, in the early Nineteenth century. Medi-Scope: The Medical Journal for Students of Medicine and Surgery in Malta, 1986, 9:18

[52] T. Chetcuti. Sulle manie. Il Filologo Maltese, 10ᵗʰ February - 30ᵗʰ March 1841

Scarificators simply made numerous small wounds prior to applying a cupping glass.[53]

In 1842, case presentations describing the management of puerperal sepsis record the use of leeches in Maltese patients in addition to formal venesection. In the first case leeches were applied on two occasions - 15 to the hypogastrium and, five days later, 24 to the abdominal wall. In the second case leeches were applied to the hypogastrium and right iliac fossa on four occasions, the number of leeches applied ranging from 18 to 50 animals.[54] Another recorded use of leeches was described in 1843. This was in a case of abdominal pain caused by intra-abdominal bleeding. This was managed by the application of 24 leeches to the painful site.[55] The use of bloodletting with the application of leeches to the temples in cases of puerperal convulsions was discussed in the Maltese medical press in 1871. While the prevalent British school of medical thought believed that venesection and the application of leeches in cases of eclampsia was without benefit and was likely to augment the convulsion, the author discusses the possible role of the procedure in cases when the mother is plethoric especially in the presence of pulmonary oedema.[56]

In 1840 the Civil Hospitals in the Maltese Islands were using 2600 leeches per month. To control the excessive consumption of these animals, instructions were issued to the medical officers to resort more frequently to cupping, as was generally practiced in the British Military Hospital.[57] The situation was apparently similar in the British Naval Hospital. In his review of cases treated at Bighi Naval Hospital during 1842-44, T. Spencer Wells apparently generally resorted to bleeding by cupping in his general

---

[53] A scarificator is in the holdings of the Our Lady of Mount Carmel Asylum Museum. C. Savona-Ventura. Mental Disease in Malta. Malta: ASMMH, 2004, 47

[54] Considerazioni teorico-pratiche sulle febbri puerperali. Il Filocamo. Giornale Medico-Scientifico e di Educazione. 1842, 2(2):17-23

[55] S. Arpa: Di un caso particolare di gravidanza extra-uterina. Malta: G. Camilleri, 1843, 7

[56] G. Gulia. Ostetricia. Sulle Convulsioni Puerperali. Il Barth. Gazzetta di Medicina e Scienze Naturali. 1871, 3(1):45-48

[57] M&H Arch. Letter from G. Montanaro to G. Casolani dated 19th December 1840. Letters from Purveyor of Charitable Institution 2nd January 1838 to 28th April 1842, fol.99-100 [manuscript held at the National Archives Museum Ms.no.84].

management. He however did resort to the application of leeches in at least six cases, generally in the management of inflammation and associated swelling and pain. The cases included: acute pneumothorax, purulent pericarditis, perforating injury of the knee joint, spinal injury causing displacement of dorsal vertebrae, ascending middle ear infection, and tubercular infection of the arm.[58] In 1851, Santo Spirito Hospital, with an average population of twenty-five patients, was using 300 leeches per month. In June 1855, directions were issued to the employees at the Central Hospital with a view of preserving the leeches for more than one application. The practice of keeping them in wood ash was discontinued. They were instead washed with fresh water after falling off from the patient, and a pinch of salt placed onto their mouths.[59]

Instructions about the application and the post-use care of leeches were similarly given by Prof. S.L. Pisani, Professor of Midwifery and Gynaecology at the University of Malta and Head of the Clinical Department of the main civil hospital in Malta, in his lectures to midwives published (in Maltese) in 1883. The lectures were originally delivered about ten years previously. In his instructions, Pisani advises that the site of application should be clean and odourless. The leeches were to be removed from their container, dried in a cloth and applied to the indicated site. This was likely to be the abdomen, while the number to be applied was generally about two dozen. If the number of leeches to be applied was numerous, they were to be applied four at a time on each side of the abdomen. After engorging themselves and releasing from the patient, they were placed in a container containing wood ash and left until they digested the engorged blood.[60]

---

[58] W. Martin, T. Spencer Wells. Report of Cases treated in the Royal Naval Hospital, Malta. Edinburgh Medical and Surgical Journal, 1844, vol.LXI(159):350-390; T. Spencer Wells. Report of Cases treated in the Royal Naval Hospital, Malta, in 1843 and 1844. Edinburgh Medical and Surgical Journal, 1846, vol.LXV(166):1-24

[59] M&H Arch. Memorandum from the Office of Charitable Institutes and Prisons, Valletta dated 22nd June 1855 to Medical Officers of the Central Civil Hospital, Santo Spirito and Gozo. Central Hospital Correspondence 16th May, 1850 to 8th December, 1858, fol.55/5 [manuscript held at St. Vincent de Paule Hospital]

[60] S.L. Pisani. Ktieb il Qabla. Malta: P. Debono & Co., 1883, 86-88

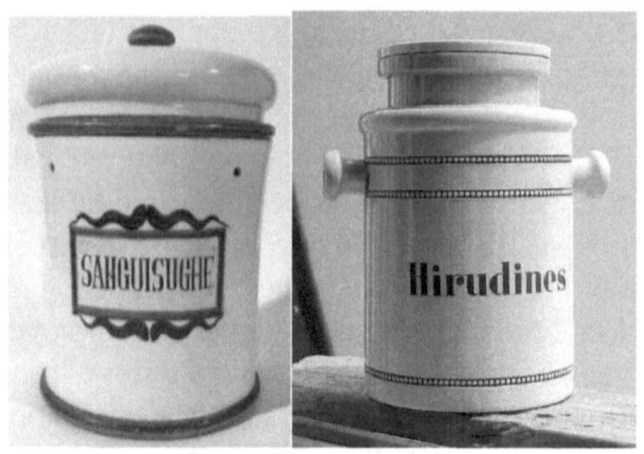

Leech Pharmacy jars

During the nineteenth century, the leeches used in the Maltese charitable institutions were purchased after a public call for tenders was issued. The contractor, who had to submit a sample of fifty leeches before being awarded the contract, bound himself to supply the quantity required for a whole year.[61] Before acceptance from the contractor, they were examined and approved by the Senior Physicians and the pharmacist.[62] Whenever allowance was made for British Military personnel to be admitted to the Civil Hospitals, the Military authorities were obliged, excepting in cases of urgency, to provide the required medicines including leeches. On the 19th March 1853 the Inspector of Charitable Institutions instructed the Resident Assistant Physician at the Central Civil Hospital that while "It is understood that the Military are to provide their own Medicines and of course leeches are included, but in case of

[61] Il Portafoglio Maltese, 3 June 1844, p.2694

[62] M&H Arch. Memorandum from G. Montanaro dated 17th December 1840. Letters from Purveyor of Charitable Institution 2nd January 1838 to 28th April 1842, fol.98 [manuscript held at the National Archives Museum Ms.no.84]; M&H Arch. Letter from G. Montanaro to E. Bonavia dated 28th June 1841. Letters from Purveyor of Charitable Institution 2nd January 1838 to 28th April 1842, fol.138 [manuscript held at the National Archives Museum Ms.no.84]; M&H Arch. Letter from Dr. G.V. Portelli Inspector Office of Charitable Institutes and Prisons, Valletta dated 21st June 1858 to Drs. Pisani, Engerer, and Ghio. Central Hospital Correspondence 16th May, 1850 to 8th December, 1858, fol.1858/22 [manuscript held at St. Vincent de Paule Hospital].

urgency you are to supply all articles, Medicines or instruments which may be required by the Military Medical Men".[63]

A late 19th century British-made pocket surgical instrument kit included an artery forceps, trocars, probe directors, scissors, bistouries or scalpels, lancets, suture needles, and a pestle. This set would have enabled the performance of minor surgical procedures including the excision of superficial tumours, drainage of abscesses or hydrocoeles, management of sinuses, suturing of lacerations, venesection and facilitate smallpox vaccination. It would also have allowed for the preparation of ointments, etc.[64]

The therapeutic option of venesection and the application of leeches continued into general use well into the early twentieth century, even after the advances made in physiology, microbiology and pharmacology. A manual for nurses published in the vernacular in 1904 still instructs these paramedical personnel on the application of leeches. The nurses were advised that the site where the leeches were to be applied should be first washed with soap and warm water, and then dried. The leeches were to be first washed and then dried with a soft towel. The animals were generally applied directly to the skin. However, a better method was to apply them by the simple expedient of overturning the jar containing the animals and some water over the skin. When this did not work, the skin could be spread with some honey or sweetened milk. In the presence of a high fever, the leeches should be "primed" by washing them in warm water. Care was to be taken whenever the site indicated for the application of the animals was close to the nose or any other orifice, to prevent them making their way into the orifice. This could be achieved by the use of special glass tubes that prevented them from escaping or by the use of a string threaded through the leeches' rear end. The leeches could be made to dislodge prior to their becoming engorged by sprinkling some salt over them. The same leeches

---

[63] M&H Arch. Letter from J. M. Collings Office of Inspector of Charities dated 19th March 1853 to Dr. P. Montanaro Resident Assistant Central Civil Hospital. Central Hospital Correspondence 16th May, 1850 to 8th December, 1858, fol.54/4 [manuscript held at St. Vincent de Paule Hospital]

[64] C. Savona-Ventura, J. Thake. Pocket Set of Surgical Instruments. It-Tabib tal-familja – Journal of the Malta College of Family Doctors, 1997, 12:2-4

could be used repeatedly on the same patient, but nurses were advised never to use the same leech on different patients. The leeches were to be stored inside a well-aerated container containing water. After use the animals were to be wetted with salted cold water and then placed in their container. [65]

The use of leeches in medicine in Malta continued to be popular in the first decades of the twentieth century. The barber-surgeons or *barberotti* remained responsible for venesection well into the 19th century and were only removed from the list of medical practitioners in 1921.[66] Until the 1930s, the animals could be purchased from a shop in the rural village of Qormi in Malta. The use of leeches apparently persisted into the 1940s.[67] Venesection in small repeated quantities was regularly used in the management of fevers; while in the presence of wounds, the procedure was believed to reduce the inflammatory reaction by helping the absorption of extravasated blood from the tissues. The procedure was also used to prevent the development of pregnancy eclampsia, cerebral stroke, and in the management of severe headache, pulmonary oedema, mental disease and gastric symptomatology. Venesection was generally performed on the jugular or brachial veins, rarely from the veins of the leg. It was sometimes combined with cupping to help extract a larger volume of blood. Leeches were also applied to reduce superficial inflammation at wound sites especially after plastic surgery such as rhinoplasty. This concept has been re-adopted in modern medicine using the anticoagulant injected by the leech to help with improving the circulation after plastic surgery.

Other folklore treatment based on rationalization was also incorporated in Maltese medical folklore. The use of poultices as emollients aimed at softening hardened skin conditions like corns. Rough skin was managed by an ointment made from beeswax melted in boiling oil. Warts were managed by applying the sap of the Tree Spurge [*Euphorbia sp.* – Maltese: *Tengħud tas-Siġra*] or of the Fig tree [*Ficus carica* – Maltese: *tina*]. These substances are believed to act as emollients

---

[65] S. Galizia, 1904: op. cit., 84-100

[66] Second Sanitary Law. Malta Government Gazette supplement. 13 May 1921, 126

[67] C. Savona-Ventura, R.T. Sawyer, P.J. Schembri. The Medicinal Use of Leeches in Malta. Malta Medical Journal, 2002 14(1):48-52

74

softening the wart allowing it to fall off. An alternative traditional medicine is to use cautery using a burnt olive twig tip and bringing it close to the wart without actually touching it. The treatment is repeated until the wart shrinks away. Other folklore treatment for skin conditions included the use of almond oil or the seeds of castor oil tree [*Ricinus communis* – Maltese: *siġra tar-riċnu*] rubbed on the scalp in cases of Cradle Cap (seborrheic dermatitis) in infants. Summer heat rash was managed by rubbing cucumber [*Cucumis sativus* – Maltese: *ħjara*] slices on the area or simply by swimming. Barber's rash was managed by rubbing the skin with a half-reduced boiled extract of the Tulliera plant [*Dittrichia viscosa* – Maltese: *tulliera salvagga*]. One further refrained from shaving for a week. Ringworm was managed by covering the area with split green immature carob pods [*Ceratonia siliqua* – Maltese: *siġra tal-ħarrub*], or dissolved mother of pearl in lemon juice, or simply with ink. A fungal infection of the lips was treatment by rubbing the lips with kerosene. A lotion made up of rum and castor oil or the fat of the ocellated skink [*Chalcidis ocellatus* – Maltese: *xahmet l-art*] was said to help to improve hair growth.[68]

Reptiles on the Maltese Islands have long been associated with the medical folklore. The advent of St. Paul to the islands in 60 ACE and the story of how he survived being bitten by a snake[69] led to the attribution of miraculous therapeutic properties for the cure of poisonous snake-bite to items such as fossil shark teeth [tongue of St Paul], fossil fish vertebrae [serpent eyes], powdered Malta rock especially that dug out of St Paul's grotto in rabat; and the saliva of persons born on the feast of the conversion of St Paul [25th January]. Other reptilian-related medical folklore is the preparation of a soup made for the local Painted Frog [*Discoglossus pictus* – Maltese: *zring*] given to sick children, or the use of fresh tortoise blood in the treatment of jaundice and epilepsy. Male jaundice sufferers were asked to bleed a female tortoise from the leg and make the sign of the cross with the blood on the joints of the arms and legs. Female sufferers were to use a male tortoise. Epilepsy sufferers were to drink the blood of a tortoise preferably after a fit. The wall Gecko [*Tarentola mauritanica* – Maltese: *Wizgha*], because of their warty-like

---

[68] G.G. Lanfranco, 1980, op. cit.
[69] Acts of the Apostles, 28:1-6.

skin, were believed to result in the development of warts and associated with leprosy.[70]

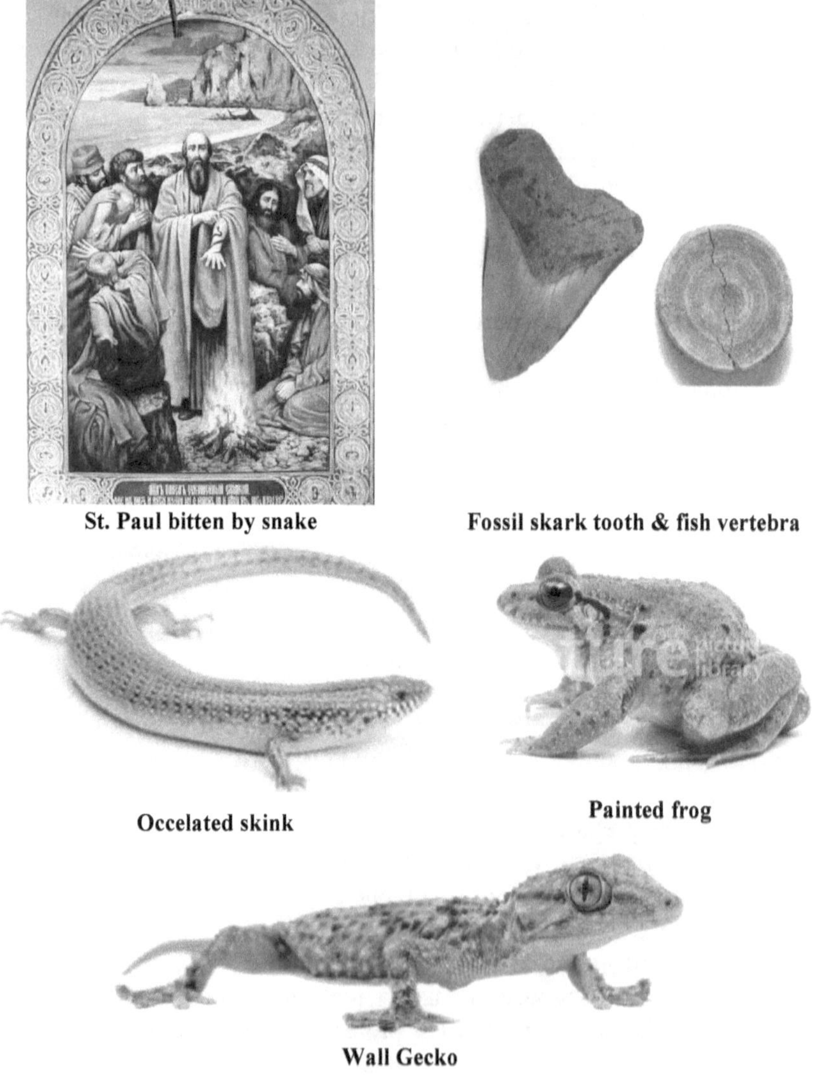

St. Paul bitten by snake

Fossil skark tooth & fish vertebra

Occelated skink

Painted frog

Wall Gecko

---

[70] C. Savona-Ventura. Reptiles and amphibians in Maltese Medical folklore. Civilization 1983; 1:258-259

76

To manage problems with postpartum breast engorgement, midwives advocated the use of a puppy applied to the woman's breast to relieve the engorgement and soften the breast to allow the child to breastfeed. A puppy placed on the abdomen was also considered useful to manage abdominal cramps – an observation recorded by Pliny in the first century ACE who recommended the use of the Maltese terrier as an ideal canine variety.

Pathophysiological evidence-based medicine

Galenic Medicine was to dominate medical practice right through the centuries until the modern concepts of physiology and microbiology were identified allowing for an understanding of the pathological process of different disease states. However, the Renaissance Period which commenced in the fourteenth century initiated a cultural movement that promoted appraisal of knowledge through a combination of reasoning and empirical evidence. In the early Renaissance, science and art were intermingled, with artists such as Leonardo da Vinci making observational drawings of anatomy based on medical dissection and observational anatomy. The willingness to question long-held beliefs, promoted by the Protestant Reformation initiated in 1517, led to the realization that the humeral theory of Galen did not always match everyday observations. The willingness to question previously held truths and search for new answers resulted in a period of major scientific advancements chemistry and the biological sciences.

In 1543, Andreas Vesalius (1514–1564) published his anatomical corpus *De humani corporis fabrica libri septem* which redefined anatomy presenting a careful examination of the organs and the complete structure of the human body based on human dissection. A detailed knowledge of anatomy allowed for the development in surgical procedures, though these were still limited in scope because of the risks of sepsis and unavailability of effective intraoperative analgesia.

Advances in defining the pathophysiology of disease states were however slower to develop. While the Renaissance and the Reformation had started the "enquiry" movement where previously held concepts were questioned on the basis of careful patient observation, the complete break from the Galenic Humeral Theory of disease had to wait the physiological advances of the nineteenth century. The Galenic Humeral Theory was replaced by the concept of the alteration of the *milieu intérieur*, a phrase coined by Claude Bernard in 1854. Bernard summarized his concept stating that: "The fixity of the milieu supposes a perfection of the organism such that the external variations are at each instant compensated for and equilibrated.... All of the vital mechanisms, however varied they may be, have always one goal, to maintain the uniformity of the conditions of life in the internal environment.... The stability of the internal environment is the condition for the free and independent life." The medical services of the Maltese Islands during these important centuries were managed by the hospitaller Order of St John that promoted a "state of the art" medical and social service system for the community. The doctors serving the community received a medical education locally and overseas ensuring that the medical community remained cognisant to developments on the mainland. Even after the expulsion of the Order of St John by Napoleon Bonaparte in 1798, Malta established political and cultural links with Britain ensuring that the medical community remained cognisant with developments in medical concepts.[71]

Other aetiological concepts were developed throughout the eighteenth century. These included the Miasmic Theory or *"mal aria"* for infectious disease based on the observation that certain infections were more prevalent where bad odours were present [odours reflecting decomposing biological material]. This was later in the nineteenth century to be replaced by the Microbial theory of infectious disease. The concept that corruption of air could contribute to ill-health was believed in Malta since the Medieval Period being referenced in the 1231 Constitutions of Melfi and subsequent *bandi* issued throughout the Medieval and Early Modern Periods.[72] The Commission of eight knights

---

[71] C. Savona-Ventura. Knight Hospitaller Medicine in Malta [1530-1798]. Malta: PEG Publ., 2004; C. Savona-Ventura. Contemporary Medicine in Malta [1798-1979]. Malta: PEG Publ., 2005

[72] J.M. Powell. The Liber Augustalis or Constitutions of Melfi promulgated by the Emperor Frederick II for the kingdom of Sicily in 1231. New York: Syracuse univ. press, 1971, 132.

sent to Malta by the Order of St. John prior to taking over the islands, reported that Malta was subject to contagious fevers particularly in month of August attributed to the fact that the inhabitants were in the habit of soaking hemp in the marshes.[73] This observation probably encouraged the Grandmaster of the Order of St. John to issue on the 23rd July 1538 the Public Health Ordinance pertaining to the washing of hemp.[74]

A similar concern occurred in August 1724 when a commission of five doctors led by the *Protomedicus* G. Zammit was set up to address whether the dirty foul-smelling waters that had collected in a garden in the vicinity of Marsamxett were injurious to public health. Again, in September 1754 when a *"fever"* outbreak devastated Mdina and its environs, a commission set up to investigate the outbreak attributed it to the fouling of the air in the region caused by the water vapours animating from the surrounding fields and gardens under cultivation.[75]

An episode of voiced concern over industrial pollution was made in August 1642. An enterprising businessman Pompeo de Fiore applied to the Grandmaster to be granted a site outside Valletta in the vicinity of Sarria for his pottery-making workshop. The reason given for this request was that the fumes given off by the kilns would have a deleterious effect on the environment. The application was forwarded to the Commissioner of Works who with the engineer Francesco Bonamici visited the site and proposed a site facing the *"tower of the fountain"* away from the fortifications of Valletta.[76]

Reference to the potential harmful effects of miasma was again made following the 1780 earthquake damage of the Church of Porto Salvo in Valletta. Since reconstruction of the church was going to necessitate exhumation of the graves, the Council of Order of St John appointed a

---

[73] T. Zammit. The water supply of the Maltese Islands. Archivum Melitense, n.d., 7:p2

[74] NLM. Universita` 13 (23.xii.1538) 162-163v

[75] P. Cassar. The concept of air pollution is over 2000 years. The Sunday Times, 15th August 1993, 34-38; NML AOM 1187, f.53 as reported in P. Cassar: Three Medical biographies. Joseph Zammit, Gabriele Henin, Joseph Edward Debono. University Press, Malta, 1984, 11

[76] NML. AOM 1184, f.326

commission to investigate the matter. This concluded that the disturbance of the *mal aria* could constitute a grave danger to public health and proposed that church burials should be abolished. To replace the mephitic gases extruding from the graves and replace this with wholesome air, the commission proposed the digging of ventilation shafts and the lighting of tarred wood to purify the air.[77]

In 1801, an epidemic outbreak of "fever" at Mdina caused alarm in the community who commissioned an investigation by the medical staff of *Santo Spirito* Hospital. In their report the physicians attributed the epidemic to the poisonous emanations in the air arising from the stagnant waters behind the city, the concentration of which had risen because the valley behind Mdina was not sufficiently ventilated to allow dissipation.[78]

The main source of harmful emissions that gave significant cause for concern was sewage. The Order of the Knights of St. John in 1569 promulgated *capitoli* that ensured that each house in Valletta was to be supplied with sewage tanks or *pozzi neri*. These were linked to the main street-drain and discharged into the sea. Similar subterranean channels were constructed in the Three Cities. The sewage disposal system resulted in the Grand Harbour becoming polluted with an effluent that gave an offensive smell which permeated into the residential areas. These exhalations were further contributed to by the numerous ventilation shafts of the public sewers. These were sufficient to blacken silver articles in houses in Bormla.[79] The sewers were constructed of porous material without reference to sectional area or inclination. They were not regularly flushed with water so that they were not cleaned or cleared of the deposits.[80]

The diffusion of the "miasmic" exhalations was blamed for the occurrences for all forms of illness. In 1865, the Chief Police Physician

---

[77] Vicq d'Azyr. Rapport sur plusieurs questions. Malta, 1781; G. Vivenzio. Risposta a molte quistioni proposte alla Societa' Reale di Medicina di Parigi. Napoli, 1781

[78] NLM. Universita` Manuscript 183, fol.53 and Universita` Manuscript 192, n.p.

[79] Il Barth, 6th March 1875, 490

[80] J. Sutherland. Report on the Sanitary Condition of Malta and Gozo with reference to the Epidemic Cholera in the year 1865. London, 1867, 44

Dr. A. Ghio opposed the "miasmatic" theory of the propagation of cholera, but he still held the view that "several other bodily disorders, especially those which appeared to consist primitively and chiefly in a dissolution of the blood, seem also to be occasioned by the continual inhalation of irresistible odours". The effluvia arising from drains were considered to "affect the composition of the blood of those who continually breathe them".[81]

In 1858, the authorities contemplated the introduction of a water carriage system of drainage for the towns. This suggestion was supported in 1867 by Dr. J. Sutherland and Captain D. Galton who had been commissioned to study the sanitary conditions of the barracks and hospitals in the Mediterranean stations. The report recommended the substitution of the drainage system with impervious glazed pipes of suitable dimensions, the trapping of all street gratings, and the provision of special arrangements for flushing and ventilating the main sewers to prevent the emission of sewer gases.[82]

Of course, not all attempts at rationalization for the causation for disease followed the correct path. The aetiological causation of congenital malformations had long been associated with superstition and in the seventeenth century, the belief was prevalent that malformations were the result of the female copulating with animals or the devil. In 1647, 17-year old Gertrude Navarre accused herself before the Inquisitional Tribunal of having had carnal relations over the previous six years with men and animals brought to her by the devil. She became pregnant and procured an abortion on a number of occasions.[83] In the 1749, the Maltese physician Dr. Salvatore Bernard adhered to the theory that the fantasy organ of the pregnant woman communicated by means of the animal spirits with the fantasy organ of the baby so that any perception aroused in the mother's mind produced a similar impression in the foetal brain, which impression

---

[81] A. Ghio. The Cholera in Malta and Gozo in the Year 1865. Malta, 1867, 19,30

[82] D. Galton, J. Sutherland. Report on the Barrack and Hospital Improvement Commissions on the Sanitary Condition and improvement of the Mediterranean Stations. London, 1863, 85; J. Sutherland, 1867: op. cit., 44

[83] A. Bonnici. Maltin u l-Inkizzjoni f'nofs is-seklu sbatax. Malta: Klabb Kotba Maltin, 1977, 102-104,199-200

in turn reacted upon and molded the form of its body. He held that monsters having the shape of animals and devils were born to women who during gestation had been exposed to the sight of these creatures.[84] These beliefs remained ingrained in Maltese mentality until relatively recent times and many congenitally malformed individuals were kept hidden away from view by their families. A special hazard of pregnancy was the emergence of longings or desires that could not be satisfied. According to popular belief, the new-born will bear the brunt of a birthmark resembling in form and colour the object of the unfulfilled desire. If a person neglects to satisfy the wishes of a pregnant woman, he/she would be punished by suffering from a sty.[85] Dr. Francisco Butigiec in 1804 did not share the notion that "in an alteration of imagination which affected the foetus in such a way as to produce a defective baby or a monstrosity".[86]

---

[84] P. Cassar. The Neuro-psychological concepts of Dr. S. Bernard. Scientia, 1949, 15:29

[85] J. Cassar Pullicino. Studies in Maltese Folklore. Malta: University Press, 1992, 213-215; P. Cassar. Pregnancy and birth in Maltese tradition. Chestpiece, 1975, 25

[86] F. Butigiec, 1804: op. cit.

Pharmacotherapy

The symptomatology of disease required supportive manage while the natural healing process took its course. This supportive management was often based on some form of pharmacotherapy generally utilizing herbal medicine. Rational medical thought also required recourse to purging using emetics or laxatives to restore the balance in body humours. The therapeutic option of purging the body from altered humours required pharmacological agents that could be used as emetics or laxatives. These were often derived from plant sources identified by observational studies noting the effects on the body system when these plants were ingested by animals or man himself.

The identification of plants as potential useful supplements in medical management was generally based on direct observational experience linking the plant with some action though experience or experimentation, or alternatively through the "doctrine of signatures" whereby a use is identified through association with the shape or colour of the plant.

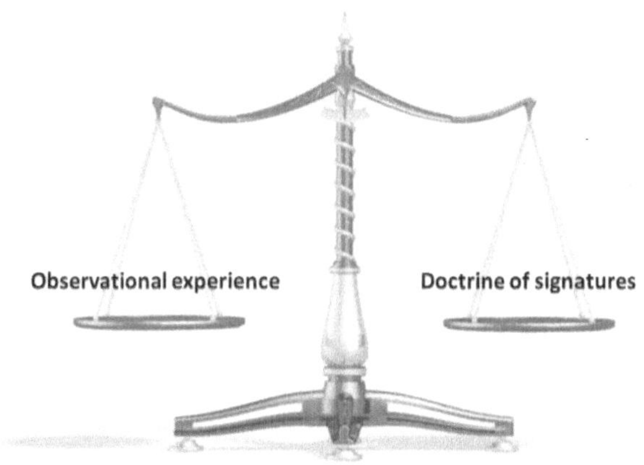

A number of medicinal plants with emetic and laxative effects have been identified to grow on the Islands. These include: the Garden Iris [*Iris germanica* – Maltese: *Fjurduliż ikħal*] which has emetic, purgative, and diuretic properties; the White mignonette [*Reseda alba* – Maltese: *Denb il-ħaruf abjad*] which has laxative and diuretic properties; the Italian lilac [*Melia azedarach* – Maltese: *Siġra tat-tosku*] with purgative and vermifuge properties; the Mediterranean buckthorn [*Thamnus alaternus* – Maltese: *Alaternu*] with purgative properties; the Sweet violet [*Viola odorata* – Maltese: *Vjola*] having laxative properties; and the Fig [*Ficus catica* – Maltese: *Tina, Farkizzan, Bajtar ta' San Ġwann*] which has a mild laxative effect while its sap can be useful for the treatment of warts and other skin conditions.

Another identified useful plant in the management of diabetes mellitus is Fenugreek [*Trigonella foenum-graecum* – Maltese: *fenugrek*] which has been identified to have metformin-like effects. [1] A number of other herbs are generally known to have a beneficial effect positively affecting for a high number of bodily functions. Because these plants add a tasty overtone to food, they are often used as an integral part of recipes. A number of herbs are indigenous to the Maltese Islands. Perhaps the most commonly known herb is Mediterranean Thyme [*Thymbra capitata* – Maltese: *sagħtar*] found growing in the wild in rocky, arid places such as stone steppes, garigue land, the coast, and within valleys. The plant is today legally protected. Thyme can be used to complement a number of recipes and sauces, and can also be drunk as a herbal tea. Studies have shown that thyme lowers blood pressure, boosts the immune system, and can be used as a cough remedy. Sage [*Salvia fruticosa* – Maltese: *Salvia ta' Sqallija*] also grows in rich soil, roadsides and valley sides. It is known for its medicinal properties being useful to manage coughs, the cleaning of ulcers and sores, rheumatism and excessive menstrual bleeding.

---

[1] J. Borg. Descriptive flora of the Maltese Islands including the ferns and flowering plants. Government Printing office, Malta, 1927

Another well-known herb that grows commonly in the wild is Common Fennel [*Foeniculum vulgare subsp. vulgare* – Maltese: *Bużbież*] found growing on dry soils around the coast. It's highly aromatic and its dried seeds are used in a number of Maltese recipes. Fennel is known to be rich in Vitamin C, fibre and potassium, reducing inflammation and cholesterol levels, as well as aiding bowel movement. The sliced bulb is also used as an additive to salads. Similarly, the herb Rosemary [*Rosmarinus officinalis* – Maltese: *Klin*] is naturally found growing on the Maltese Islands in rocky valleys. It is generally used as flavouring for red meat, but is rich in Vitamin B and Vitamin A. It is known to be an antioxidant, being also antibacterial, anti-inflammatory, and a natural remedy for headaches and colds. The White Wall Rocket [*Diplotaxis erucoides* – Maltese: *ġarġir abjad*] belonging to the cabbage family has diuretic properties, though this is not generally used medically; however, the Star-of-Bethlehem [*Ornithogalum arabicum* – Maltese: *ħalib it-tajr il-kbir/ħarjet iċ-ċawla*] is well known for the medicinal use of its bulbs, which contain chemicals known to be of use in treatments required for congestive heart failure. A tisane of boiled flowers is said to induce a state of mental peace, calm dreams, and be a good treatment for shock.[2] To calm down the mental state, the roots of Bermuda Grass [*Cynodon dactylon* – Maltese: *Niġem*]   or boiled Lemon Verbena [*Verbena officinalis* - Maltese: *Buqexrem*] are recommended.[3]

Other plant products were identified as potentially useful against specific disorders through the "doctrine of signatures" whereby a use is identified through association with the shape or colour of the plant. One such plant in use by Maltese practitioners was the parasitic plant known as General's Root or Maltese Fungus [*Cynomorium coccineum* – Maltese: *Għerq il-ġeneral, Għerq sinjur, Żobb l-Art*]. Because of its dark red colour it was assumed to be useful in conditions involving blood such as dysentery, bloody evacuations, every haemorrhage in the chest, treating gums, hematemesis, drying wounds, and to control traumatic and surgical

---

[2] https://www.eve.com.mt/2016/09/04/native-wild-herbs-of-the-maltese-islands/
[3] G.G. Lanfranco, 1980: ibid; G. Lanfranco, 2001: ibid., 1-33

bleeding. Its phallic shape made it supposedly useful to manage venereal disease. It has now been shown to have a hypotensive effect. [4]

Since prehistoric times, man has looked to the environment and through experiential medicine identified elements in the environment that potentially may be useful to manage the symptomatology of disease and effect cure. These elements are generally derived mainly from plant products, but incorporate also animal and mineral components. The first list of pharmacological agents mentioned in the historical record in Malta dates to 1345 when these items had a 10 percent tax imposed upon their importation. The 19 products listed in the *Capitula Sagati* of 1345 included mainly items of botanical origin: The medications listed mainly include items of plant origin and two items respectively derived from animal or mineral origins: *jnchensu, masteca, diaculogna, risialgaru, juriulena, granata dulcj, menduli ad minutu, melj, trimintina, zaffarana, zinchiparu, cannella, grarofalj (sic! sive scarofali), cera, bolu, nuci di Jndia, cardamunj, anzarutu, sanguj di dragunj, mirra.* [5]

jnchensu = Incense	Incense is aromatic biotic material composed of aromatic plant materials that release fragrant smoke when burned. It was burnt to counteract or obscure malodorous products of human habitation and thus was used for aesthetic reasons, and in therapy, meditation, and ceremony. It may also be used as a simple deodorant or insectifuge.
masteca = Mastic resin	Mastic is a resin obtained from the mastic tree *Pistacia lentiscus*. Mastic has been used as a medicine since antiquity and was used as a remedy for snakebite, for the prevention of digestive problems and colds, for bronchitis and for improving the condition of the blood. It was also valued as a breath freshener and a tooth whitener. It is now known to have antioxidant, antibacterial and antifungal properties.
risialgaru = Arsenic	Arsenic is a chemical element that is highly toxic. In subtoxic doses, soluble arsenic compounds act as stimulants and also has been used in the management of infections such as syphilis and trypanosomiasis. It is also useful in the management of skin disorders such as psoriasis.

[4] C. Savona-Ventura. Cynomorium coccineum Linnaeus - 17-19th century Materia Medica Melitensis. Maltese Family Doctor, 2007, 16(1):p.6-8

[5] S. Fiorini. Kura u Servizzi tas-Sahha f'Malta sa nofs is-seklu XVI. In: Oqsma tal-kultura Maltija (T. Cortis, ed.) Ministry of Education, Malta, 1991, pp.233-234.

juriulena = Sesame seeds	Sesame seeds is derived from the flowering plant *Sesamum indicum*. It was included in the list of medicinal drugs in the Egyptian medical scrolls dated to be over 3600 years old. It is a common ingredient in various cuisines. It is known to have a beneficial effect on blood pressure and reduces oxidative stress markers and lipid peroxidation.
granata dulcj = Pomegranate	The pomegranate is a fruit-bearing deciduous shrub *Punica granatum*. It is generally used as a culinary item, but was used as a medicinal ingredient in many remedies for the treatment of tapeworm and other infections.
menduli ad minutu = Sweet almonds	The almond (*Prunus dulcis*) is a species of tree native to Mediterranean climate regions. The nut, especially the bitter variety, has a large amount of the poisonous hydrogen cyanide. The sweet almond has only trace quantities. Sweet almond was used as a mild laxative, and was applied to the skin to soften chapped skin, to soothe mucous membranes, and to kill germs.
melj = Honey	The honey is an animal product produced by the Honey bee (*Apis mellifera*). It was used as a sweeting agent and the produce the alcoholic drink mead. It has antiseptic and antibacterial properties and was used to treat open wounds.
trimintina = Turpentine resin	Turpentine is a fluid obtained by the distillation of resin from the pine-tree. Turpentine has been used medicinally since ancient times, as topical and sometimes internal home remedies. Topically, it has been used for abrasions and wounds, as a treatment for lice, and when mixed with animal fat it has been used as a chest rub, or inhaler for nasal and throat ailment. Taken internally it was used as a treatment for intestinal parasites, but because of its toxicity, it should never be taken internally.
zaffarana = Saffron	Saffron is a spice derived from the flower of *Crocus sativus*. While mainly used as a culinary product, saffron has a long history of use in traditional medicine. Egyptian healers used saffron as a treatment for all varieties of gastrointestinal ailments. It was also thought to be useful for wounds, cough, colic, and scabies, and in the mithridatum remedy used as an antidote for poisoning.
zinchiparu = Ginger	Ginger is the rhizome of a flowering plant *Zingiber officinale* which has been widely used as a spice and a folk medicine for conditions such as colds, nausea, pain, arthritis, migraines, and high blood pressure
cannella = Cinnamon	Cinnamon is inner bark of the tree species *Cinnamomum verum* which is widely used as a spice. It has a long history of use in traditional medicine as a digestive system aide. Recent evidence suggests that it acts as a hypoglycaemic agent and helped lower cholesterol and triglycerides.

scarofali = Cloves	Cloves are the aromatic flower buds of the tree *Syzygium aromaticum*. Clove oil has long been used in traditional medicine to manage toothache pain and other types of pain. It has also been used as an antiseptic, anti-fungal, antibacterial, antioxidant, analgesic, and anti-inflammatory. Their use is recommended to treat coughs, flatulence, inflammation, tooth aches, and bronchitis.
cera = Wax	Beeswax (*cera alba*) is a natural wax produced by honey bees of the genus *Apis*. Beeswax has mild anti-inflammatory effect and has been used to reduce inflammation, manage ulcers, and treat diarrhoea and hiccups.
Bolu = Medicinal clay	Various varieties of clay have been used in traditional medicine being used by the ancient Egyptians. Its external application is useful to manage skin conditions; and internally to soothe an upset stomach or as an anti-diarrhoeal medicine.
nuci di Jndia = Nutmeg	Nutmeg is the seed or ground spice of *Myristica fragrans*. In traditional medicine, nutmeg has been attributed with health benefits including that of promoting digestion, supporting oral health, detoxifying the body, supporting kidney health, treating insomnia, relieving pain and treating cancer. Other benefits included treating inflammation, promoting blood circulation, supporting immune system, treating acne and delaying aging. Nutmeg has no known medicinal value and in high doses intoxication may occur inducing delirium, anxiety, confusion, headaches, nausea, dizziness, dry mouth, eye irritation, or amnesia.
cardamunj = Cardamom spice	True Cardamom is a spice made from the seeds of the plant *Elettaria cardamomum*. It is used for digestion problems including heartburn, intestinal spasms, irritable bowel syndrome, diarrhoea, constipation, liver and gallbladder complaints, and loss of appetite.
Anzarutu = Arum plant	Arum is produced from a common woodland plant species *Arum maculatum*. The root has been used for nutritional and medicinal purposes for many centuries, despite their toxicity. They have been used to manage colds and swelling (inflammation) of the throat. It is also used to promote sweating and to loosen chest congestion.
sanguj di dragunj = Dragon's Blood Tree resin	The dragon's blood was collected from the plant *Dracaena cinnabari*. In the Mediterranean basin it was used as a dye and in medicine as a sort of cure-all – used for general wound healing, a coagulant, curing diarrhoea, lowering fevers, dysentery diseases, taken internally for ulcers in the mouth, throat, intestines and stomach, as well as an antiviral for respiratory viruses, stomach viruses and for skin disorders such as eczema.

| *mirra* = Myrrh | Myrrh is a natural gum or resin extracted from a number of small, thorny tree species *Commiphora myrrha*. It is used as an antiseptic in mouthwashes, gargles, and toothpastes; and also, is used in some liniments and healing salves for abrasions and other minor skin ailments. Myrrh gum is commonly claimed to remedy indigestion, ulcers, colds, cough, asthma, lung congestion, arthritis pain, and cancer. |

Mention has already been made of the use of a number of indigenous and imported plant species to manage external and internal medical conditions. Decoctions were particularly important in the management of internal disease. A decoction of the Bermuda Grass rhizomes [*Cynodon dactylon* – Maltese: *Niġem*] is reportedly useful to 'purify the blood', to alleviate hypertension, to promote a diuresis, and to manage breathlessness. A decoction of a mixture of boiled plants made up of Bermuda grass, Vervain, Pennyroyal, Mint and Maltese Savory [*Satureja microphylla* – Maltese: *Spakkapjetra*] was supposedly useful to manage jaundice.

Puryfying blood	<ul><li>Bermuda Grass rhizomes decoction</li><li>Parsley decoction</li><li>Mallow leaves decoction</li><li>Fumitory decoction in milk</li></ul>
Hypertension	<ul><li>Bermuda Grass rhizomes decoction</li><li>Olive leaves decoction</li><li>Eating of raw garlic with bread</li><li>Cumin and Vervain decoction</li></ul>
Diabetes	<ul><li>Lemon Verbena decoction</li><li>Endive decoction</li><li>Spiny Chicory decoction</li></ul>
Jaundice	<ul><li>Mix of Bermuda grass, Vervain, Pennyroyal, Mint and Maltese Savory decoction</li><li>Squirting cucumber juice placed near nostrils</li><li>Horsetail decoction</li></ul>
Gallbladder problems	<ul><li>Horsetail decoction</li></ul>

Kidney stones	<ul><li>Maltese Savory decoction</li><li>Maize fibre with an orange split into three and sugar decoction</li></ul>
To stimulate diuresis	<ul><li>Bermuda Grass rhizomes decoction</li><li>Barley water</li><li>Boiled onions decoction</li><li>Maltese Savory decoction</li><li>Spiny chicory decoction</li><li>Maize fibre decoction</li><li>Horsetail decoction</li></ul>
Fever	<ul><li>Garlic with sugar and water, drinking the concoction first thing in the morning after letting it stand overnight</li><li>Thorny or Morning Star thistle infusion</li></ul>
Cough and other respiratory ailments	<ul><li>Borage infusion with/out honey or honey with lemon or milk</li><li>Carob syrup [*Gulepp tal-Harrub*] diluted as a warm drink possibly including fig or borage infusion</li><li>Southernwood infusion</li></ul>
Gastro-intestinal disturbances	<ul><li>Teas infused from various plants including mint, chamomile, laurel leaves, cloves, Southernwood, Horsetail, onion, and elder (also useful for hiccups).</li><li>Olive or almond oil, or infusion of olive leaves</li><li>Prickly Pear flower or quince decoction to manage diarrhoea</li><li>The inner threads of the pumpkin fruit are said to be useful to manage tapeworms</li><li>Senna leaves or chamomile infusions can be useful to stimulate a bowel movement in constipation.</li></ul>

Useful references:

1. To help relating English vernacular names of plants with the Maltese vernacular and scientific names refer to: Stephen Mifsud MaltaWildPlants.com, 2002-2018 go to http://maltawildplants.com/
2. For the list of protected species of animals and plants according to the L.N. 311 of 2006 ENVIRONMENT PROTECTION ACT (CAP. 435) Flora, Fauna and Natural Habitats Protection Regulations, 2006 go to http://www.maltawildplants.com/!docs/Misc/LN_311_2006_E.pdf
3. T.J. Tabone, M. Azab. Edible Wild Plants – A foraging guide to 15 common plants growing in Malta. Friends of the Earth, Malta, n/d. Part of a larger toolkit at www.foemalta.org/goodfood.
4. WHO monographs on selected medicinal plants. World Health Organization, Geneva, 1999. Available from: https://apps.who.int/iris/bitstream/handle/10665/42052/9241545178.pdf;jsessionid=1FFB0D48B9729F2E6FF82E6944621C6D?sequence=1
5. E. Attard, H. Attard, A. Tanti, J. Azzopardi, M. Sciberras, V. Pace, et al. The Phytochemical Constitution of Maltese Medicinal Plants – Propagation, Isolation and Pharmacological Testing, Phytochemicals - Isolation, Characterisation and Role in Human Health, A. Venket Rao and Leticia G. Rao, IntechOpen, 2015. DOI: 10.5772/60094. Available from: https://www.intechopen.com/books/phytochemicals-isolation-characterisation-and-role-in-human-health/the-phytochemical-constitution-of-maltese-medicinal-plants-propagation-isolation-and-pharmacological